DEMYSTIFYING MIND CONTROL
AND RITUAL ABUSE

DEMYSTIFYING MIND CONTROL AND RITUAL ABUSE
A Manual for Therapists

Alison Miller

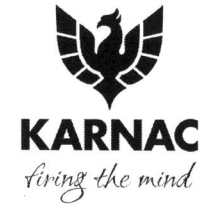

KARNAC

firing the mind

First published in 2024 by
Karnac Books Limited
62 Bucknell Road
Bicester
Oxfordshire OX26 2DS

Cover art: Artist Jen Callow says: "This picture represents our inner people and the supportive inner community we have built over the years, which has been a key piece of our healing from ritual abuse and mind control."

British Library Cataloguing in Publication Data

A C.I.P. for this book is available from the British Library

ISBN: 978-1-80013-265-8 (paperback)
ISBN: 978-1-80013-274-0 (e-book)
ISBN: 978-1-80013-275-7 (PDF)

Typeset by Medlar Publishing Solutions Pvt Ltd, India

www.firingthemind.com

Contents

About the author

Alison Miller is a retired clinical psychologist, who practised in Victoria, BC, Canada for over forty years and specialized in work with survivors of ritual abuse and mind control for the last twenty-five years. She is the author of *Healing the Unimaginable: Treating Ritual Abuse and Mind Control, Becoming Yourself: Overcoming Mind Control and Ritual Abuse,* and (with Wendy Hoffman) *From the Trenches: A Victim and Therapist Talk about Mind Control and Ritual Abuse,* and has contributed to various edited collections and journals.

Preface

This book is written for the person I was in 1990, when I met my first ritually abused client and desperately sought for help in understanding what I was dealing with and knowing what might help her. It is for every therapist who is now in that situation.

Even if you are a highly experienced therapist, you are facing something new when you see your first victim of childhood mind control. You may still develop a strong therapeutic connection with your client. You may still find the techniques in which you have been trained helpful. But these clients are unique in that their minds have been coopted for the purposes of organized criminal groups. They have not just been abused, they have been abused in systematic ways to produce the behaviors the abusers desired. Everything you have learned so far will still apply, but you need more. You need to understand what your client has gone through and the most effective ways to counter that and set your client free to take charge of their own life. This book attempts to provide that information.

The following quotation from Harvey Schwartz is from an online discussion of the Organized and Extreme Abuse discussion group of the International Society for the Study of Trauma and Dissociation (ISST-D) posted May 1, 2019.

> Demystification is essential to our work. If therapists do not know or understand the specific methods, madness and dynamics of organized perpetrator groups including mind control, bizarre but strategic set-ups, lethal twinning, patterns of interlocking lethal double binding and variations on coerced perpetration … our patients will be insidiously abandoned (without professionals treating them even realizing it) to their own dissociative worlds of internalized domination, annihilating shame, and soul murder. And their heartbreaking spirit-crushing isolation will be reinforced without anyone ever realizing this. Then, patients' acting out, retreat, or other mysterious behaviors in therapy might be misrecognized by ill-informed, or limited informed therapists who may end up frustrated and perhaps even acting out their helplessness and frustration on the patient, further reinforcing the pathological belief systems installed by the perpetrators and cultivated in years of living hell.
>
> It is so important for our field to educate the larger trauma and mental health field about what survivors have actually lived through, as well as the what and how of the machinations of the perpetrators so therapists' minds and hearts can stretch to provide the kinds of holding, witnessing, containment and demystification necessary for healing extremely malevolent trauma. More than anything it is essential to realize that traumatized patients will not reveal to us or themselves, these extremely bizarre and sadistic experiences if they do not sense that we have some ability to "go there." And, more than that, an ability to willingly and courageously go there with them, but to go there with a combination of compassion, ferocity, and acceptance.

Introduction

In 2012, I published *Healing the Unimaginable: Treating Ritual Abuse and Mind Control*, a book that has provided a basic understanding for many therapists working with victims of these atrocities. I have been delighted to see that the contributions of the survivors I have known, both through their own writings in that book and to my own understanding, have helped so many therapists and survivors. Since that book was published, I have learned more about how such abuse works within the brain of the victim, and how these abuser groups work. In 2022, five years after my official retirement, I presented a ten-session webinar series on treating survivors of organized extreme abuse featuring ritual abuse and mind control, hosted by the non-profit organization Survivorship. The webinars are available at https://survivorship.org/survivorship-webinar-2022-healing-the-unimaginable-a-ten-session-course/.

At the end of the course, one participant described the series as "a distillation of much of the content in *Healing the Unimaginable* with an emphasis on the practical." He said that the webinar series struck him as a step-by-step guide to working with survivors of ritual abuse and mind control, looking at "how to work with/do XXX," "how to manage XXX," and "what to do if this or that happens." He concluded that "A book which provides information in a format similar to the lecture series would be a valuable reference guide for therapists and a helpful companion piece to *Healing the Unimaginable*."

So, here is that book. This book is not a new edition of *Healing the Unimaginable* and is not a substitute for that book, which is not out of date and covers the topic in depth, including invaluable contributions from survivors. But hopefully this new book will fill a need for therapists who need a succinct, practical, down-to-earth guide for this challenging work.

Many therapists feel unqualified to treat these complex clients, and try to refer them on, but there is a desperate need for therapists who will rise to the challenge. This book will help you understand what you are dealing with and how to approach each situation.

In this book, I race through complex and difficult topics. All the way through, I invite you to consider that we are talking about human lives here, the immensely difficult and challenging lives of our clients, people whom we would have been if we had been born into a different family.

CHAPTER 1

Dissociation, ritual abuse, and mind control

Organized abuser groups have discovered that they can train their victims to cooperate with the abuse, forget what has happened, and maintain the security of the abuser group. They accomplish this through the creation of severe dissociation in the victims.

Dissociative splitting

In infancy or very early childhood, when a child is exposed to severe trauma, especially if that trauma is repeated, especially if it comes from caregivers, and especially if is inescapable, dissociative splitting occurs. My theory of how it works is based on what survivors have told me that organized abuser groups knowingly do to children for the purpose of creating new identities within children. A child's conscious awareness is contained within a particular brain circuit. When severe trauma occurs, the circuit in use becomes overloaded and a new circuit takes over consciousness, while the traumatized circuit is put into "storage." I call this dissociative splitting. Dissociative splitting affects survivors' awareness of some or all of the traumatic events, the circumstances surrounding the events, and the identity of the abusers, for some period of their lives. It is a biological adaptation that enables a child to live with ongoing trauma, in many or most cases involving his or her own parents or caregivers. Once this has happened, it is possible for a child to have one part who believes the parents are kind and caring people, and they have a normal life, and another part who endures the ongoing abuse. What I am talking about is unimaginable harm done to an innocent infant by people who are supposed to take care of that infant.

Diagnoses

The mental health field is full of diagnoses, as if by naming something and listing its characteristics we have captured the essence of what a person is going through and can now fix it. For a long time, the dissociative disorders were not recognized, and sufferers were saddled with labels like bipolar, schizophrenic, and borderline, and treated with medication rather than with compassionate care. But the wheel has turned, and mental health professionals have begun to recognize the existence of mental disorders caused by trauma. The U.S. National Child Traumatic Stress Network states:

> "Complex trauma" is a relatively new term which is used to describe both children's exposure to multiple traumatic events— often of an invasive, interpersonal nature—and the wide-ranging, long-term effects of this exposure. These events are severe and pervasive, such as abuse or profound neglect. They usually occur early in life and can disrupt many aspects of the child's development and the formation of a sense of self. Since these events often occur with a caregiver, they interfere with the child's ability to form a secure attachment. Many aspects of a child's healthy physical and mental development rely on this primary source of safety and stability. (https://hrsa.gov/behavioral-health/national-child-traumatic-stress-network-nctsn)

The poor attachment between the child and parents is the basic situation that enables the dissociative splits, like the fault in the earth that enables earthquakes. Complex trauma usually gives rise to a dissociative disorder in the child. When there are specific parts of a person who "come out" into the world separately, have their own histories, and are often amnestic for what happens when other parts are in control of the body, mental health professionals call it dissociative identity disorder (DID). This term has replaced multiple personality disorder (MPD). When parts do not take control of the body in everyday life but there is evidence of their internal presence, we call it other specified dissociative disorder (OSDD). All survivors of extreme organized abuse, especially ritual abuse and mind control, have one of these conditions, whether or not they are aware of it. One of my first such clients taught me that these conditions should be looked at as mental injury rather than mental illness. Persons who suffer from them are not "crazy." The conditions usually begin in infancy because of severe and ongoing neglect and trauma, and such people grow differently because of the repeated injuries.

For simplicity, I shall refer to people with both these conditions as "multiple." This acknowledges their internal experience, so I shall use this term even though the label "multiple personality disorder" has gone out of fashion. And I'll call those of us who do not have split minds or brains "singletons," acknowledging both our continuity of identity and our inability to escape the full impact of our experiences through dissociation.

Organized child abusing groups deliberately try to split and structure their victims' minds in such a way that they will not remember what happened, or that if they begin to remember they will disbelieve their own memories. Their goal is OSDD, a victim who is multiple but does not appear so, so that the deliberate trauma is not suspected. The deliberately created inner parts come out upon instructions or triggers by perpetrators rather than spontaneously.

The website of the International Society for the Study of Trauma and Dissociation (ISST-D.org) has in its member resources section some excellent guidelines for work with persons experiencing DID. I recommend that all persons treating ritual abuse or mind control survivors become familiar with those guidelines. My approach follows those guidelines but goes beyond them with information and treatment recommendations specific to survivors of these most horrific and deliberately planned abuses.

Ritual abuse and mind control

Organized abuse

Michael Salter (organisedabuse.com) states that organized abuse involves multiple adults who conspire to sexually abuse one or more children. Organized abuse can include the sexual exchange of children between perpetrators as well as the production and distribution of child sexual abuse material. This definition focuses on the sexual abuse rather than the more extensive torture employed by ritualistic and mind-controlling abuser groups, of which sexual abuse is an important part but far from the whole thing. Sexual abuse, including production of child sexual abuse material to be distributed online, is one important funding source for organized perpetrator groups, which may have entirely different long-term goals, including political ones.

The Center for Knowledge on Transgenerational Organized Violence in the Netherlands (https://kenniscentrumtgg.org/what-is-organized-abuse/) distinguishes three groups or networks who engage in what they call "transgenerational organized violence":

- Family or transgenerational networks: adults who as children were abused themselves by a network and who now abuse their own children or allow them to be abused.
- Groups that are linked not by family ties but by the ideology or purpose of the group. The abuse takes place in groups. Children are "recruited" in daycares, schools, churches, and through other social groups. Women within the group also give birth to children that they hand over to be abused by the other members of the group. These groups can last many generations.
- Ad hoc groups: people who come together to form a new group with new ideologies and rituals.

They point out that ritualized abuse can include physical, sexual, mental, and emotional abuse, and that victims and survivors are programmed to silence. They allude to ideology, which I believe is important, as the larger organized groups (such as modern-day Nazis) as well as the religious (primarily Satanic or Luciferian) groups have an ideological basis and goals. It is all organized evil.

Mind control

Mind control is a primary objective (and methodology) of those orga-nized groups who systematically abuse children. I define mind control as abuse of children (and adults) by an organized group that deliberately creates, indoctrinates, and trains internal parts (alter personalities). Beliefs are implanted and parts trained through deprivation, torture, electroshock, drugs, and stage magic to do "jobs" for the perpetrator group. This is much more than organized sexual abuse.

I realize there are other forms of mind control; for example, the mind control of entire populations by such methods as controlling the media so people hear only what the authorities want them to hear. But the kind of mind control I am talking about is central to what these organized groups do. Whether their aim is simply to maintain secrecy while mak-ing a lot of money from child trafficking and the production of child sexual abuse materials, or to indoctrinate a huge number of children in order that the perpetrator group will take over the world, the method is the same. The community of therapists treating complex trauma and dissociative disorders and researchers investigating organized abuse need to be clear about the importance of mind control. These abuser groups plan out their victims' personality systems, keep records of all the parts they create and the jobs they assign to those parts, provide internal accommodation for the parts within the brain of the victims, keep records of everything they have done, and maintain their security through torture and threats to their victims at all ages.

Programming

Certain persons within organized abuser groups have the job title of "programmer," and attempt with some success to program victims' brains. It is true that people are not nearly as predictable as computers. But we know that the brain contains many circuits with both electri-cal and chemical connections. And the deliberate splitting of parts in infants appears to rely on the way this circuitry works. Electroshock is a primary methodology in training. Our brains are vulnerable, especially in infancy. There is only one way to create persons who can engage in spying, sex slavery, assassination, or ritual murder without any con-scious awareness of this when not engaged in these activities. The way is through abuse and torture of small children, separating parts of their minds that are then indoctrinated and trained individually as the abusers see fit. I have known several brave survivors who have nevertheless overcome their programming and become free and outspoken warriors for justice.

Survivor therapist Arauna Morgan has defined programming (of people) as follows: "Programming is the act of installing internal, pre-established reactions to external stimuli so that a person will automatically react in a predetermined manner to things like an auditory, visual or tactile signal or perform a specific set of actions according to a date and/or time." Some people object to the use of this term, but I use it because it is used by the perpetrators, and it unfortunately describes what those perpetrators are attempting to do.

Groups who engage in mind control

I have heard of several groups who engage in this type of mind control. They include:

- Military or political groups (such as some within the CIA, MK-Ultra, Nazis, KKK, Russian and Chinese intelligence)
- Traditional organized crime (child prostitution, child pornography, drug couriers, assassination, placing members in political office or positions of power)
- Religious groups (Satanists, Luciferians, Setians, Black Santerians, Druids, ancient religions, new religions). See Stella Katz's descriptions in *Healing the Unimaginable*, p. 93. These groups often consist of multigenerational incestuous families who traffic their own children. Michael Salter's recent research suggests that law enforcement needs to pay more attention to the role of such families in child trafficking. It is not clear whether all such families belong to occult religions.
- Secret societies (such as Illuminati and some within the Freemasons—occult/political conspiracies).

The groups are interconnected. A person who has been trained by one abuser group is likely to have training by other groups as well. There are training centers who will train (that is, torture and abuse to produce particular results) children for different groups who request it. The late Stella Katz (a pseudonym), who contributed a lot to my understanding of how all this works and wrote an important chapter in *Healing the Unimaginable*, worked as a programmer of young children at such a center.

Some of the major organized perpetrator groups believe in the importance of bloodlines. Only people with the proper bloodline (such as descendants from some of the early leaders who developed the methodology and goals of the group) can rise to power in such groups, and those designated to be kings or queens or other leaders are required to take such leadership and are severely punished if they refuse.

Ritual abuse

I define ritual abuse as mind control by a religious group. There are well-organized perpetrator groups whose religion involves sacrifice to a deity such as Satan and Lucifer. Although Satanic trappings (costumes etc.) are used for the purpose of frightening child victims in pornographic settings, there are also genuine evil religious groups. Others who have worked in this field define ritual abuse as any abuse done in a ritualized repetitive manner, whether or not religious.

Recognizing a survivor client

These checklists are provided in my self-help book for survivors, *Becoming Yourself: Overcoming Mind Control and Ritual Abuse* (2014). They are reproduced here for therapists.

Some mind control indicators

- Your client has been diagnosed with DID or OSDD (although it is important to note that although these conditions do come from severe early trauma, not everyone who suffers from them has experienced mind control).
- Your client hears voices or thoughts ordering them not to talk or to be quiet (which means they have been ordered by abusers not to talk

about the abuse, which may or may not be organized abuse involving mind control).

- If your client talks about what may have happened to them, they experience symptoms like bodily pain, nausea, a severe headache, spasms as if receiving an electric shock, or flashbacks of violent events. (This kind of reaction is quite likely to indicate the presence of programming, internal parts doing the assigned "job" of giving the symptoms if the survivor disobeys orders.)
- Sometimes your client feels that there is something foreign inside their body that can do harm to the client or others (a lie they were told as a child).
- Sometimes your client feels that there is something foreign inside their body that can signal their location or thoughts to abusers (another such lie).
- Your client has unexplained scars on their body or scars with a nonsensical explanation. (This indicates at least severe trauma that is not remembered because of dissociation.)
- Sometimes your client feels that their energy will poison those they are close to (yet another lie told to the child).
- Your client worries that they will harm or murder someone or that they have done so. (Particularly in ritual abuse, a victim is forced to participate in abuse and/or murder in rituals and then told that they are evil because they did this.)
- Your client is preoccupied with or needs to avoid newscasts, articles, or conversations about ritual abuse or mind control. (This preoccupation may indicate that the client is wondering about whether they have experienced these abuses and/or that they have been ordered not to acquire information about such abuses.)
- Your client is unable to look at you. (This may indicate anti-therapy programming: see Chapter 2.)

Some ritual abuse indicators

- Your client has made drawings characterized by ritual-like features, such as a lot of red and black, knives, fire, cages, robes, body parts, blood. Children draw what they cannot speak, and adult victims have child parts.

- Your client has worse psychiatric symptoms around their own birthday, family members' birthdays, Christmas, Easter, Halloween, May Day, and early September. (These dates are common times when rituals occur.)
- Your client has cut patterns, symbols, or letters on their own body. Many trauma survivors use physical pain to push away emotional pain, but the presence of patterned cuts can indicate parts following instructions, and the patterns give revealing information.
- Your client finds odd, ritualistic songs or chants running through their head, sometimes with a sexual, bizarre, or "you'd better not tell" theme. (Abusers teach such songs and chants to children, for later use as reminders to remain loyal. Nursery rhymes are also used, with special meanings for survivors.)
- Your client has intrusive thoughts or impulses regarding violent sex, sex with children, sex with animals, or sex with corpses. (Ritualistic groups do these things, as do many organized perpetrator groups involving these extreme kinds of child abuse.)
- Your client's dreams and/or flashbacks include rituals. This kind of dream does not occur spontaneously to people without such a background, although horror movies can temporarily have such an effect.

Indicators—fears and phobias

There are many fears and phobias that may indicate such abuse, as these are experiences that have been traumatic for survivors of these abuses. Of course, some of these may indicate other traumatic experiences, such as family members getting drunk on Christmas.

- Birthdays and weddings
- Religion and church
- Christmas and Easter
- Doctors, dentists, hospitals
- Injections and needles
- Bodily fluids and excretions
- Red meat and/or certain other foods
- Cameras and being photographed
- Specific colors or shapes

- Harm being done to your loved ones or your pets
- Ropes, being tied up, being hung
- Confined spaces, basements, crawl spaces, pits, cages
- Death and burial
- Weapons
- Police, jails, and cages
- Baths and drowning
- Insects, snakes, spiders, and rats
- Discovering that they are a perpetrator.

Qualifiers of indicators

- Some of the fears (like needles or insects or the dentist) are common. If your client has these, do they have a way to account for them in their life history?
- Other fears on this list, and the non-fear items, are uncommon. Does your client experience any of the uncommon ones? Do they have a way to account for them in their life history?
- If you gave your client the list of indicators to check off, look at the entire pattern of the client's answers. No single one of these items means a person has a history of ritual abuse or mind control. However, if they say yes to a large number of them, you might suspect such a history.

(Thanks to Pamela Reagor, Catherine Gould, and Ellen Lacter for earlier lists.)

Remembering the abuse

Training not to remember

For the most part, survivors of these abuses don't remember most of their abuse. Dissociation blocked the front parts of the child from that knowledge and continues to do this even when abuse is ongoing in adulthood. Training by perpetrator groups makes survivors unaware of their dissociation by creating "walls" between the front parts and the inside parts and using memories of antipsychotic drugs to suppress internal voices. Important training experiences are surrounded with a barrier of torture, electroshock, pain, spinning, and drugs (before and after) that are reexperienced if such a memory is to be accessed. And parts are trained so that if a survivor remembers anything, they will immediately remember the threats made to them about the perils of disclosures and may also remember being an apparent perpetrator.

In addition, the perpetrators design experiences that will discourage remembering. For example:

- Perpetrator group members waken and abuse a child at night, then a parent responds to the child's distress by telling the child that nothing happened; it must have been a dream.
- Parents take a child to a simulated ritual murder of someone known to the child. The next day the child sees the apparently murdered person alive, speaks about the event, and is told they must have imagined it.
- The groups stage implausible scenarios, such as alien abductions and abuse by people dressed as cartoon characters, aliens, demons, or celebrities. Parts of the child are ordered to make the person remember these things if they start to have abuse memories.
- The parents take the child to a "hospital," where a "doctor" simulates an operation to place a bomb apparently in the child's belly. The "hospital staff" show the child an X-ray of a body with a bomb inside it and say, "If you tell anyone about what we do, this bomb will go off inside your body."
- The abusers put a small animal, such as a rat or a snake, in the child's vagina or anus and tell the child that telling anyone about the abuse will cause that animal to eat them up from the inside.
- Another simulated operation places a supposed recording device in the child's body and the "doctor" tells the child that this device will tell the abusers if the child tells any secrets.
- The abusers use trickery, such as plastic ears glued to a wall, or apparent eyes on a wall or stuck to the back of a mother's head, to make the child believe that the abusers see or hear everything they say or do. An inner part of the child is instructed to make the survivor see these (memories) if they are tempted to talk about the abuse.

Abuser groups offer adult survivors incentives, such as family love or money, to recant what they have disclosed. Everyone wants to be loved by their family, and many survivors are poor, so these incentives can have a strong effect, keeping survivors out of therapy or at least preventing them from making any disclosures. Like scammers, these abuser groups will figure out what lure works for which victim.

How parents discourage children from remembering

Parents in these perpetrator groups are instructed to respond to disclosures with:

- "You made up all those things you think you remember."
- "You have a vivid imagination. Those things aren't real."
- "It was a dream. You can't tell a dream from reality."
- "You got those weird ideas from TV programs/the internet/something you read/someone else's experience."
- "That crazy therapist is putting ideas into your head. You should go to a therapist but not the one you have."
- "If you 'see' awful things, those are dreams/your vivid imagination/ signs that you are crazy."
- "If you hear voices, it means you are psychotic and should be hospitalized." (Unfortunately, much of the psychiatric profession agrees with this.)

"Do you believe me?"

Our clients frequently disclose something outrageous, then ask us "Do you believe me?" To a therapist, this feels like a double bind. You're damned if you say you do believe your client, as you can be accused of encouraging the client in inventing things. You may be inviting a lawsuit regarding suggesting false memories. And you're damned if you don't say you do, as the sincere client feels invalidated. So how do you handle this question?

"Therapeutic neutrality" versus reflective belief

Ever since the late 1980s, when therapists first discovered these abuses, we have been attacked for believing our clients. An approach called "therapeutic neutrality" has been recommended. In 2019, I had a debate with Colin Ross in the online journal *Frontiers in the Psychotherapy of Trauma & Dissociation* about this. Ross had written an article giving an example of his supposed therapeutic neutrality. In the article he suggested saying to a self-identified ritual abuse survivor, "I don't believe you and I don't disbelieve you. I believe in therapeutic neutrality." After I read Ross's article, I asked a dissociative survivor with whom I worked for many years what she would have said if I had told her this. She responded that she would have said, "Thank you for your time. Goodbye." She would have felt disbelieved and unsupported. That client was more polite than many would have been.

Ten years earlier, Onno van der Hart and Ellert Nijenhuis wrote a wonderful article on this topic. Here are some quotations from this article:

> Clinicians should not reflexively accept or reject as fact a client's initial report of uncorroborated abuse. However, by maintaining a neutral stance, clinicians may fall short of therapeutic honesty and transparency, may fail to promote reality testing, and may not perform the necessary step of bearing witness to the client's victimization.
>
> Persistent therapeutic neutrality often becomes problematic for the client, the therapist, or both. This approach ultimately may make the client feel doubted or, worse, may be experienced as actively malignant if it is felt to represent a repetition of the negation of his or her selfhood by victimizers. How could it not be perceived this way? The failure of others to bear witness to the clients' victimization and suffering can have devastating consequences for their ability to heal. (1999, p. 37)

They quote Laub regarding Holocaust survivors:

> This loss of the capacity to be a witness to oneself ... is perhaps the true meaning of annihilation, for when one's history is abolished, one's identity ceases to exist as well ... It is the encounter and the coming together between the survivor and the listener which makes possible something like a repossession of the act of witnessing. This joint responsibility is the source of the re-emerging truth.

They recommend that therapists "should delay forming a belief about the validity of reported memories of trauma," but "develop a reflective belief in collaboration with their clients" (p. 38).

Responses to "Do you believe me?"

When asked "Do you believe me?" I prefer to say something like, "I'm a psychologist, not a detective. I wasn't there when your traumas happened. My job is to support you in making sense of it all. It is *your* life, and it is up to *you* to decide what is real by listening to all parts of yourself."

I am also aware that organized perpetrator groups engage in a great deal of complicated deception. So I say something like, "There is a difference between believing that bad experiences happened, and believing what your child parts were led to believe. It will be your job (not mine) to figure out what's real, what's unreal, and what may be a result of abusers' deceptions."

These statements empower the client in taking back control of their life. There is no need to make a point of one's neutrality, even though some therapists do this for self-protection or bowing to peer pressure, at the expense of the therapeutic relationship.

Wait for the evidence to emerge

You don't have to decide immediately about to what extent you believe what your client is telling you. Be careful not to suggest things, while remaining aware of what could be going on. Respond to disclosures with empathy and with confidence, letting the client know you can handle such disclosures. Don't get caught up in the false memory controversy but stay with the client's experience. Your client is likely to disbelieve their own memories. Do not focus on memories initially but explore the personality system and inner world before exploring the traumatic memories. That will come later. When everything seems to fit together—the symptoms, the story, the life circumstances—over time we can come to reflective rather than reflexive belief.

CHAPTER 2

The therapeutic relationship

I have always believed that the therapeutic relationship is the essential ingredient in psychotherapy. Without a strong therapeutic bond, therapy for almost any condition will fail. Knowledge and techniques are less important than the relationship. If you have never worked with these survivors before, be assured that if you are able to develop a healthy therapeutic bond, you can acquire much of the knowledge you need from your own client, despite all the client's training not to tell.

But of course, you can save a lot of time and mistakes by learning what those who came before you have discovered. My first book, *Healing the Unimaginable: Treating Ritual Abuse and Mind Control* (2012a), gives a lot of detail about ritual abuse and mind control, and has many valuable contributions from the survivors I have known. With your survivor client, you can go through my workbook for survivors, *Becoming Yourself: Overcoming Mind Control and Ritual Abuse* (2014). I have heard that survivors of these abuses are ordered not to read that book. *From the Trenches: A Victim and Therapist Talk About Mind Control and Ritual Abuse* (2018), which I co-authored with survivor Wendy Hoffman, is a collection of essays on this topic. I do recommend you read these, as this present book is a simple summary of ideas that are drawn out in detail in those previous books.

Anything may be the presenting problem when a survivor comes to therapy—whatever your previous specialty is. One of my first four survivor clients came for parenting issues (my previous specialty), another for "schizophrenia" involving flashbacks of ritual abuse, another for sexual perpetration against her younger brother, and the last for severe long-term depression with suicidality. When I look back on past clients from the time before I knew about dissociative disorders or ritual abuse (the 1980s and early '90s), I recognize two others (both diagnosed with bipolar disorder) who were probably survivors of this abuse, and my survivor clients told me of two other former clients of mine (an anorexic teen and an indigenous woman with parenting issues) whom I did not recognize as survivors of such abuse.

A victim may come to you because of fragmentary memories of extreme abuse that the client doesn't know whether to remember or believe. Or it may be a first awareness of multiplicity within: hearing voices, messages from parts, etc. Victims of these abuses often go to therapy because they are commanded to go to a "plant" therapist, one who secretly works for the abuser group, who will have the capacity to close down their memories and discourage them from significant healing work. Some clients who come to you may have already spent some time with such a therapist.

Underneath the surface of any presenting problem, the client is assessing you to see whether you can handle what they need to tell someone and whether they can trust you.

The therapeutic bond: parental and infant love

A 2012 pilot study of 163 professional therapists by Adah Sachs found that therapists had different boundaries with dissociative clients than with other clients. 85% of those therapists she studied did so. They felt that these boundary changes were necessary parts of their duty of care. The modifications of boundaries included offering time outside normal working hours, outside the office, and during therapists' holidays. They risked themselves professionally and personally. They said such things as: "This case, I don't even take to supervision." The more experienced and qualified therapists made the most modifications, and among the professions, psychiatrists and medical doctors made the most modifications. There was a high burnout rate among these therapists.

My hypothesis is that dissociative clients, who have infant parts, elicit parental love from therapists, and it is this parental love that creates a particular kind of bond with our dissociative clients. The victim clients feel love for you if they are finally able to tell their story and have someone actually listen, rather than dismissing their concerns.

The bond between parents and babies is one of the strongest forces in nature. Parents are hardwired to love their babies. As a mother's due date nears, her brain starts producing more and more oxytocin, a switch that turns on parental instincts. As she holds, rocks, or nurses her baby, she gets a rush of dopamine, the main currency of pleasure in the brain. Fathers too feel some of these changes. Any parent knows the wonderful enthrallment of being with this new little person.

This is what happens to an attuned therapist when we encounter a highly dissociative client for the first time. We fall in maternal or paternal love with the client because we sense the unbonded infant parts who desperately need this bond. But most of us don't understand what is happening. We may think it's romantic love. Or we may want to adopt the client as one would adopt a child, add this person to our family. I have heard of many therapists who did this kind of thing in the early days of DID therapy. Larry Pazder, who wrote the book *Michelle Remembers*, the first book about ritual abuse, married his client. The client too may be confused, when very young parts fall in infant love with the therapist as with a nurturing parent, and want to be held or hugged, despite the terror of other parts. Adriana Green's heartbreaking story "Downfall" (2014) describes how it felt to a highly dissociative client when her therapist misunderstood the love between them and overstepped her boundaries. Sometimes those infant parts offer themselves sexually, as that is what had to happen at home.

Farber (2018) suggests that therapists experience a "dissociative attunement" that activates the client's internal infant's symbiotic fantasy of being one with the good mother, as

> the analyst's attuned unconscious receptivity … makes possible
> a form of human experience not quite like any other, through
> sharing elements in common with other relationships of intense
> resonance, intimacy, care, vulnerability and mutual personal

and interpersonal knowledge … The therapist must become a microtonal tuning fork, having a dissociative attunement that is an implicit knowing.

The term "dissociative attunement" refers to the fact that an attuned therapist is attuned to parts of the client who are not immediately visible. This attunement is often something we are aware of, something that guides our therapy. We become aware of parts who are present, almost as if we can see them behind the client's eyes. We modify the way we speak to our clients on the basis of things we intuit, such as which parts might be present. We make comments like "I think someone else is listening. Is there something they'd like to say to me?" We dream about our clients. I dreamed the name of one client's system leader part, which she hadn't told me, and an important part of the primary structure (internal design) of another client's system, which she hadn't yet told me.

The relationship is mutual. The babies within the dissociative client glom onto us, like a baby glomming onto the mother. They yearn desperately for the "good enough mother" they never had. The strength of the attunement, the parental and infant love, is what carries us through all the enormous ups and downs of the long-term therapy process.

The vulnerability arising from hurt infant parts leads us to fall in maternal/paternal love with them. We want to be constantly there for them and protect them, and we may easily let go of our boundaries in this process. The neglect and constant boundary invasion they have received leads them to want nurturing like little babies. They are insensitive to their own and others' boundaries because they are babies, and they were never permitted to have boundaries in their families. It is easy for a therapist to become enmeshed with such a client, especially if we have never worked on developing firm boundaries ourselves. Out of love, we promise what we can't deliver. This leads to eventual abandonment of these clients. Several of my long-term dissociative clients came from therapists who had abandoned them after promising the moon. Survivors' child parts expect sexual abuse, and some are trained to seduce therapists. Perpetrator groups will command that seduction in their effort to invalidate any therapy that might help. A therapist's misunderstanding the feeling of love can lead to serious ethical violations.

Many of us therapists do love our clients, and this enables that attunement that allows us to perceive their needs and their strengths. As we tune in to what is going on in them, the relationship grows into one of mutual respect and trust. The love between us carries us through the ups and downs of the therapy process.

How abusers try to prevent the therapeutic bond

Mind controllers know the importance of the therapeutic relationship because it is where the secrets of the client's abuse might be disclosed. They go to extra trouble to make sure such a bond never happens, or if it does happen, that it will be disrupted and broken. They forbid their victims to have any bond of love with anyone. They assign victims their "friends" and their spouses, making sure that love does not happen.

Destroying the bond with the victim's mother

Abuser groups give pregnant women victims electric shocks that cause them to leave the fetus emotionally. After the child is born, the abusers test, through such things as pin pricks, to see whether he or she will accept comfort, because if the newborn does, he or she is not programmable and may be killed. Mothers who are victims are not permitted to bond with their children. There is severe neglect and deliberate breaking of potential bonds. Each mother is made to walk by her screaming infant, paying no attention to the child's suffering or hunger. Parents, both male and female, are ordered to sexually abuse their children, and they do it in fear that the children will be killed if they don't.

Training not to form bonds

The following are ways I have found that child victims are trained not to form loving bonds.

- Cult parents give their children animals to pet and love, and then the animals are killed, with the children being forced to hold the weapon that kills the pet, and even if they refuse, they are blamed for the death. There are forced choices like "Kill this rabbit or we will kill your little brother."
- A child is paired with a "disposable" (usually unregistered or kidnapped) child, given a chance to make friends with that child,

often the only friend the child has ever had, then forced to participate in the friend's murder. Sometimes it is a known child who is
then said to have died of an illness, with a cooperative doctor to sign
the death certificate. This is an important event in the life of most
victim children.

- The children are told that if they love someone, that person will be
  killed.
- If a child begins to form a loving or trusting relationship with someone, that person's murder may be simulated.
- If a victim has a relative or classmate who is ill or dies, the victim is
  told it was his or her energy that caused this to happen.
- A child in need of help is forced to choose for that help between
  people in hooded robes or people in ordinary clothes. If she chooses
  the ordinary looking ones, they abuse her; the robed ones are nice
  to her.
- A child is allowed to build trust with someone who turns out to be
  an abuser.

So, don't be surprised when your client has difficulty forming a bond
with you. The client may be fearing that this bond will get you killed
or that you will turn out to be a perpetrator.

Training not to trust therapists

Child victims are given specific training to believe therapists are going
to be abusers. In many cases, a child is taken to a "therapist" (who may
or may not be a real therapist) and told not to look at him. After some
time, he tells the child to look at him. Now he is wearing a devil mask
and horns, and he rapes the child. I have heard this from several survivors. The perpetrators tell children that any therapist they talk to will
sexually abuse them.

The message repeated thereafter is "Never look at therapists."
This sets the scene for later impersonation of genuine therapists who
might help. Pay attention if your client won't look at you. A woman
came to me for a consultation to figure out whether she had programming. Her inability to look at me was one of the important signs
I recognized.

Another kind of staged therapy session for children has the therapist lock up the child in what appears to be a mental hospital, where the child is drugged and abused. Afterwards the parents say, "If you show physical evidence or tell of the abuse to any professional, that person will not believe you and will lock you up forever in a mental hospital where you will be drugged and abused."

Another scenario has an apparent therapist gain the child's trust by listening and trigger a disclosure from the child by a signal to tell all. Then other perpetrator group members show up and punish the child severely, telling the child that therapists are all members of the group and will report everything the child says to the group leaders. Parents also say, "Therapists' only purpose is to get you to disclose the secrets of our group, which is strictly forbidden and extreme disloyalty to the only family you will ever have."

Another trick of abuser groups is to use words frequently used by therapists such as *feel*, *touch*, *safe*, *free*, *light*, and accompany those words with torture, so that any therapist the victim subsequently consults will be likely to use such trigger words and see the client react with terror. In addition, if a therapist uses the term *alter* personality, it may remind a survivor of *altar*, the table upon which sacrifices are made. There are also techniques therapists use that have been appropriated by perpetrators for their own goals: hypnotic induction techniques, EMDR-like movements, and especially touches used in kinesiology. If you normally use any of these things, make sure they will not be triggering for your client.

Dissociation makes it possible for parts who go through these training experiences to send their fear to other parts who do not have conscious memories of the deceptions.

Impersonation of therapists

For us therapists, there is something worse than simulating our words and techniques: We may be impersonated. Members of the abusive groups study therapists by attending their lectures, becoming their clients briefly, or sending a client in to a session with a recording device. They observe what clothing we wear, what we smell like, and all the intonations of our voices. They find a way into our office or use another space that resembles it. Then an actor impersonates us and abuses the drugged client. This happened to me with my first four survivor clients, and with at least one subsequent client. I had to get a new, more secure office with a security alarm (not purchased from the big alarm company, which had perpetrator group members on their staff). Unable to get into this new office, the abusers took a client into a nearby office with a similar layout and staged a "therapy session" in which my impersonator raged at the client but did not attack her physically or sexually. This was more successful than the physical and sexual assaults used with previous clients in deterring the client from continuing to see me, probably because it was more believable.

If you have evidence that you are being impersonated, you may want to tell your client about something unique about you (not on your face, which victim clients may not see) which is difficult to simulate. A blind part may recognize your smell and be able to tell that the abuser therapist is not you (though fragrant body products you use can of course be used by the impersonator).

Talking with someone who's multiple

I need to remind you at this point that if you have a client who is a survivor of these abuses, that client is multiple—that is, they have many hidden inside parts, most of them infants, children, or adolescents. If you are the therapist trying to help someone who is multiple, you need to learn from your client. This begins by permitting them to be your teacher about multiplicity. The first thing is to let go of the assumption that you are conversing with a single unified person. Or, if you recognize the existence of different "personalities" in the person, that they are entirely independent and need to be treated individually. Talking with a multiple is somewhat like (as in the movies) talking with identical brothers or sisters who impersonate one another, change places fast, and look the same but act differently. You need to learn to recognize the physical evidence of them changing places, and the body language and maturity level of different parts.

The front part ("apparently normal personality" (ANP)) of your multiple client may be just a "shell" who bridges the transitions so switching is not obvious, or may be a particular combination of parts who are permitted to be "out" in the body together. Do not assume the front person is the "real" person and the others less real, or that the front person can control the behavior of the other parts. Do not assume continuity of memory.

An analogy that I learned during my initial training was that talking with a multiple is like speaking with many housemates on the phone. One housemate at a time, not always the same one, can control the voice and speak with you. The house has a speaker phone so those near the phone (but not everyone) can hear you. You can talk through to others in the house. You can send messages to ones far from the phone. You can ask others in the house to give information to the one on the phone. Of course, you're not really on the phone, but you can see the person's body, and you may notice the client pauses as if listening to something other than your voice. If this happens, speak more slowly, pause, and repeat yourself, so that the part you're talking with can talk and listen to their inside parts as well as you.

All this seems obvious to me now, but frequently when I'm at a training event for therapists, I see the participants assuming the front person is more real and more important than the other parts, assuming they have continuous memory and know what is going on inside. They are nonplussed about how to communicate with the others.

It is easy to "talk through" to other parts who are listening. Just assume other parts are listening, look for evidence of their presence, and acknowledge them with kindness. And don't assume at any point that the person you are speaking with is an adult or is the usual front person. Multiples often switch and we are unaware of it.

As you get to know different parts, it is important not to show favoritism. The cute little child who is so fascinating may be distracting you from the real work, which involves dealing with the protector/persecutor parts, and many other parts who have important roles.

Detecting switches

In early therapy, most victim clients switch between parts subtly. Their language may change. The content of what they are saying may change while their voice sounds the same. A "word salad" (earlier thought to be a sign of schizophrenia) indicates rapid switching. Their emotional state may change. You can ask if this is someone new, if they know you, and if they know where they are. If you suspect it's a child part, ask the child's age so you can communicate appropriately. Do not ask their name, however, as names are used by perpetrators to call out parts they want to abuse.

Detecting co-presence

You may sense a change in emotional state. Some things you can say are, "Is someone else here?" "I sense someone is feeling scared—is that you or someone else?" Then, speaking to a part you know, "Can you tell them who I am and where we are, so they won't be so scared?" Always assume that more than one part is present. With experience, you will get to the point that you can almost see the new part behind the client's eyes.

Parts' identities

So, what parts might be within your client? Each part is very limited in its range of emotions and intellectual capacity. Most are children. Opposite-gender parts are common. Some parts may be blind or deaf or mute, often from literal responses to abusers' words ("Don't talk," "You are not seeing/hearing this, it is not happening"). Some parts may believe they are other people, like perpetrators or soldiers. Some may believe they are supernatural or alien beings: demons, ghosts, or animals. They may believe themselves to be still living in the places where their abuse happened. The inner world may be as real to many parts as the external world. Parts new to the present are often confused about time and place and date, and it's helpful to update them by, for example, showing them a calendar or something with the current date on it.

Match your style to the part(s) presenting

Interacting with a person who is multiple is a dance—you shift with their state, as you might with a baby who laughs then cries. Attunement is essential. You are often talking with an insider when you think it's the front person, the adult. See how old the person appears from their speech and body language and match your language to that age. Be assertive with tough parts, but be careful, as even a slightly raised voice can engender terror. The part you are speaking to may ask or think: "Are you going to shout? Are you going to hit me?" Some tough parts have tender ones hidden underneath the surface. Parts can themselves be multiple.

Using inner voices to establish communication with parts

Notice when the client seems to be paying attention to something internal. You can say:

- "Did someone inside say something to you? … What did they say? … Do you know what they mean?"
- "Could you ask the person who said that why they said that? Can they explain for me?"
- "Do they have any questions for me? … They can talk through you." Then,
- "Would they be willing to come out and talk to me so I can understand them better?"

Noticing subtle reactions, misunderstandings, and triggering

Watch for these reactions and address them immediately. You may ask questions like:

- "Is someone inside reacting to something I said or did?"
- "I scratched my ear because it was itchy. It wasn't supposed to be a signal to any of you."
- "Is there something in this room that makes you feel unsafe? Do you need to look around? Should I remove something?"

Watch for reactions to trigger words that have opposite meanings, such as "free" and "love." Try to avoid these words. Figure out what are trigger words for each client. Organized perpetrator groups deliberately give these words opposite meanings to those we know.

Improving inner communication

The first thing you can do is demystify multiplicity by explaining how severe childhood trauma, especially mind control programming, creates a compartmentalized brain, so people who are multiple suffer from mental injury, not mental illness. The treatment of an injury is to bring the broken parts back together, not to medicate. Your client is not crazy. Learning about the biology of dissociation helps people accept the diagnosis with dignity. Then, if they don't already know how to communicate with the other parts, you can coach them. You can frequently suggest that the client "ask inside." If they don't know what this means, you can suggest, "Just think it in your head, and then listen for an answer. It could be words, or a thought, or a picture." Then, after a few seconds, "Tell me what answer you received. Do you understand it?" If they are hearing something from inside parts, you can now enter dialogue with the insider through the presenting part. "Ask them …" It is common that insiders will say something rude or will swear. Don't be taken aback by this. The parts doing this are protectors who don't know whether you are safe to be around. Just take it in your stride. *"Ask inside" is probably the most useful thing you can say to a multiple client. Make it a habit in your dialogue with such clients.*

Relating to child parts

Usually, most parts are children of various ages, split off by horrendous events that prevented them from further life experience and growth. Young child parts have concrete and literal thinking. They may not understand words or concepts such as "lying," "then versus now," and "memory." You may or may not notice childlike grammar and thought. Find out the age of the part you are speaking with to assess cognitive maturity; talk as if to a child of that age. And remember other parts are listening and you should be clear to those ones too. Infant parts may be unable to speak and may just look at you. Don't be surprised if child parts come out and stare at you or talk to you. The internal leaders put out little ones to watch how you treat them, to see how trustworthy you are. Older parts may be able to describe what was going on when an infant part was "out" in the body. I believe child parts are still developmentally children, though not "normal" children.

Complex multi-system clients

Some multiples have very complex personality systems, with hundreds or thousands of parts. This is usually a sign of sophisticated organized abuse involving deliberate splitting off and training of parts. It's important to remember that it's all one brain. Information often reaches through barriers even when it isn't supposed to. In these cases, some deeper part of the brain holds enough wisdom to know which things to bring up, in what order. It's a system. You don't work with Susie, or Enforcer, or The Whore, for example. You work with the system.

This also applies to clients whose abuse has involved technology and other more recent inventions, such as training to control brainwaves. No matter what has been used on someone, they still have one brain whose circuitry has been disrupted by deliberately designed trauma. They are still a personality system. There is no magic in modern techniques; the abusers still rely on deliberately created dissociation, deception, and instructions to parts. And you must still rely on the therapeutic relationship rather than trying to use technical shortcuts.

Important therapist qualities for this work

You have to care, care about the child and the child parts in the adult who went through experiences of unimaginable horror. You have to be willing to expose yourself to awareness of these things, even though just hearing about it traumatizes you and makes you afraid. It is not our technical skill that makes our work effective. It is the love and caring that makes the difference, along with willingness to learn about these abuses from your client and from those therapists who have gone before you. Even when we care, knowledge about how mind control works helps us know what to say and do.

To work with clients with a background of ritual abuse and mind control in particular, a therapist needs to have patience, and be able to maintain consistency over time. Such clients have significant early trauma, and it does take years for the recovery process. They sense your sincerity, your tiredness, and your fear. They probe you for weaknesses, and they also assess your goodness, your resilience, and how much you can take if they disclose important things to you. Acknowledge your weaknesses; don't pretend they aren't there.

You need to have firm and flexible boundaries. Don't make promises you can't keep. You can't meet the infant parts' needs. You can't keep such clients safe, and multiples, especially ritual abuse and mind control victims, are often unsafe. (Hospitalization, by the way, is usually ineffective in achieving safety, even temporarily.) Therapists frequently stretch themselves too far in the effort to meet the needs of infant parts or keep their victim clients safe. I have seen therapists initially entranced with their multiple clients who then gave more and more time rather than having strong boundaries, then eventually gave up, especially when their spouses objected to the clients coming first in their lives.

You need to decide very soon whether you're going to be there for the long haul. You may feel underqualified. We all are. However, your work will improve with practice. Meanwhile, when you make mistakes, just look for opportunities to apologize. Perpetrators don't apologize. You can learn from your clients and become adept at this work, as you would with any work. It is more complex than regular therapy, and it is challenging, but it is very rewarding.

Developing the therapeutic relationship

Besides all the horrible training victims have had to discourage them from forming a therapeutic bond, we must still deal with regular old transference. Transferences onto therapists, partners, and bosses are based on previous experience through which people have developed their attachment styles. Of course, people who are multiple may have several different attachment styles within one body. So don't be surprised if your survivor client behaves in different ways towards you at different times.

Attachment styles of parts

Some parts will act out the type of attachment behavior that worked (to achieve relative safety) with their original caregivers. Some other parts will still reach out for the safe, secure attachment that might be possible with you. And you will respond. But be aware that the other parts are present. I have met several survivors who had a brief, safe, healthy attachment with someone who was in their life for a short time and then was taken away or killed. That experience nevertheless helped them realize what a safe attachment could be like, and that it is possible for them, so even if they fear the same happening to you, they will yearn for that connection, which every mammal needs in order to mature and thrive.

My very first survivor client, who came to me for parenting help, was dominated by her needy inner infants. If I'd have permitted it, she would have moved in with me. She lurked in the hallways of the mental health center where I worked, hoping to catch a glimpse of me. She even followed me into the washroom. She sought constant reassurance and expressions of affection and caring. Her neediness was smothering. She wanted much more of my time and energy than I was able to give. She was convinced I was deeply attached to her when I was actually feeling overwhelmed, confused, and irritated by her. Perhaps she knew something about me that I didn't know. I had to set firm boundaries and frequently reaffirm them. She needed a caring therapeutic relationship, but I could not parent the infants within her; her adult parts needed to learn how to do that.

When we are overinvolved, there is a risk that clients will lose their existing capacity for self-care. Although they have survived many years of abuse and neglect, their unmet need for a nurturing parent may lead them to rely on us instead of themselves whenever there's a crisis. Clients tend to commit suicide either in hospital or when just released from hospital because they have turned over to us the job of keeping them safe. (Of course, this may also be because hospitals are often not safe places for survivors of mind-controlling abuses.)

Aided by all the anti-therapy programming, your client is likely to have transference regarding trauma. Parts of your client will expect you to abuse them, emotionally, physically, and sexually, especially if they have prior experience with a plant therapist. As they were emotionally abandoned by their mother, they will expect the same of you, and since you are unable to give them the full-time nurturing attention that every child needs, they will experience your limits as abandonment.

So, they may act out in anger towards you the feelings they could not express towards their original caregivers or their plant therapists. They may accuse you of incompetence. They may challenge you and catch every error you make. Some parts may invite you into power struggles, saying very unkind things to you and trying to provoke you to be hurtful and abusive. They may engage in projective identification, trying to make you feel as helpless and worthless as they feel. No matter what you do, they may feel abandoned by you because the therapeutic relationship is time-limited and circumscribed; it cannot provide what a loving parent should have provided many years ago.

If parts have training to displace their anger (see Chapter 3), especially if they have current contact with perpetrators, they may take all the anger they have against family and perpetrators and dump it on you. This will be even stronger if the perpetrator group impersonates you. Keep in mind that the angry and hateful behaviors may be coming from parts who are just doing jobs assigned by the perpetrators. You might ask whether this is the case, and if they say yes, you could tell them that they did a fine job, and could you please speak with some other parts who might appreciate your help. You could ask the parts who hate you to talk with other parts who know you better than they do. Even after significant healing, a client may have parts with anger against you engendered by lies the perpetrators told them and may continue to tell them compounded by the natural process of transference.

Time and trust

There is no substitute for time in building trust. Your clients will watch your every move and analyze your every word to see whether you are trustworthy, believing that it is most likely that you are not, but hoping desperately that you will prove to be a person they can trust. Many survivors, however, have a developed sixth sense, and if you are trustworthy, they will sense it even if they think it is too good to be true. Take your time, and be patient with yourself, too. At the start, just deal with the presenting problem. The client will let you know when they are ready to go deeper. If they don't, and you have had some time to prove yourself, you may prod them a little. Treat all parts with consistency and fairness. When new parts emerge, they may have no sense of time. Suggest they talk with parts who have a history with you, so they can catch up on what the other parts have learned about you.

You can say, "I don't expect you to trust me. I don't trust you yet either. Trust takes time; it must be earned." They are taken aback when you say you don't trust them either, but the honesty of this statement may get through to those parts who want honesty.

You can also say, "Are you waiting for me to change? Become angry or sexual? I won't do that. The parts/inside people who protect you can watch me and see if I switch." And (if this is true), "I can't switch. There's no one else inside me. I do have emotions, which you will notice, but I can't change that much because there's only one of me."

Invite your survivor clients to ask questions. Give them opportunities to disagree with you. Tell them explicitly that you appreciate their stating their disagreement, and you accept it and won't punish them. And I repeat, apologize when you have made a mistake. This is something abusers never do. Our mistakes give us the opportunity to acknowledge our humanity and our equality with our clients.

Empathy, warmth, and genuineness

Many years ago, the research pointed to three factors that made therapy effective: empathy, warmth, and genuineness. These are absolutely basic for effective therapy with survivors of horrendous child abuse, including mind control. Genuineness means being yourself, not pretending to have more knowledge or more resilience than you actually have.

How much of your own life should you share with your clients? If you have something in common with a client, you might want to share something about this. But be careful about over-sharing. Therapy is not about you; it is about your client. And remember that dissociative people frequently have parts who transfer the anger and hatred they were terrified to express to abusers onto therapists. Such parts will use your personal disclosures for malicious purposes, especially if the client is reporting about your therapy sessions to current abusers.

Explaining your role

I imagine you have your own standard method for introducing yourself and helping your client become comfortable with you. Given the extent of the abuse these clients have suffered, however, there are additional considerations. If at some point in the early sessions, your client appears to be anxious or afraid, explain who you are and where you are. Ask if the client is afraid of you. If so, state clearly that you aren't like the people who hurt them, and they are welcome to send out their protector parts to question you. If they bring up memories, it is important to state that your role is not to force them to talk about what happened to them, but to help them heal from those events and to help them be in charge of their own life. You say this because perpetrators, anxious to maintain the security of the group, may have told them that therapists will pressure them to reveal the group's secrets.

If your client seems afraid but denies being afraid of you, you might ask, "Who outside you knows what we talk about?" If your client has made it clear to you that they were abused in this manner, you might ask directly: "Are you scared the abusers/your parents/the mean guy will know you talked? How will they know? Who will tell them? I won't. Will some part of you tell them?" (There are likely to be reporter parts inside whose job is to tell the abusers what happened in therapy.) If the client states that the abusers know by magic, or new sophisticated technology, etc., you want to address the BIG LIE, which is that the abusers know everything the person says or does or even thinks (see Chapter 3).

Your office rules

Quite early, it is helpful to state the rules of how to behave in your office. These were my three simple rules:

1. Don't hurt people
2. Don't break things
3. Don't take clothes off (except coats and boots).

Tell your clients that the rules apply to you as well as to them. This gives some reassurance you may not abuse them. These clients understand rules. They haven't had the experience of the rules applying to the other person too, but it may be both surprising and reassuring to hear you say this. In my opinion, most other rules are unnecessary. These rules are simple enough that child parts can understand them.

Guidelines about boundaries

Your relationship with your client is not confined to the time spent in your office. You need to work out a set of explicit boundaries and stick to them. Issues of trust will arise no matter where the boundaries are placed, but the boundaries do help.

These clients are desperate for connection, and once past the initial fear, some of them want to move in with you. They want your constant availability. Giving in to this understandable desire ignores our real human limitations, leads to increasing dependence on us, and fails to prepare clients for real life. Some survivors are trained to burn you out with increasing demands. But if you set clear limits on this, the parts in charge of it will respect you and respond to you.

I find one ninety-minute session per week can work well, though I've also done planned "intensives" with several hours per week for a speci-fied length of time to resolve a particular problem. You need enough time in a session to have discussion with parts who are not out front at the start of the session.

Set clear limits on contact outside of therapy sessions, such as emails, phone calls, and texts. If you say you'll only respond in a crisis, some clients (or their handlers) will manufacture crises. If your client is one who keeps trying to find a way to have more contact with you, it may help to leave the client a little recorded message each week that they can listen to instead of initiating direct contact with you (although there is always the possibility that an abuser may emulate your voice and leave a message purporting to be you). One of my survivor clients kept getting messages from "me" canceling our appointments, and she had to check with me to see whether they were genuine.

Touching

Hugs are a natural way to express affection for your clients. It may be abusive to never touch people who have been so massively neglected and abused. But with people for whom sexual abuse was the norm in all relationships, it is important that you do not touch in any way without explicit permission. Always ask permission of the part who is present so that part can set their own boundaries, and ask also if it is a problem for any other part. If you detect a sexual response in the client, discuss it openly and state explicitly that you will not be sexual with any clients, that it is against the rules for therapists. Permit your client to hug you if it feels appropriate and not intrusive. You can model good boundaries in this respect. One male client of mine struggled with whether to allow his part called "the horny goat" to be present when I hugged him. He finally concluded that this part desperately needed a non-sexual hug even though it was in a permanent state of sexual arousal.

Be aware that your client may have been told that they will poison anyone who touches them. So always ask permission. Sometimes holding a client's hand is all that they will tolerate.

Commitment and money

Working with a client with this history is a long-term commitment. Do not take them on unless you know you want to and are able to follow through. Many such clients have very little money. Do not start with anyone who cannot pay anything unless there are very special circumstances. If funding runs out, it is not ethical to just terminate the client. Do not allow the client to owe you money. Negotiate payment clearly at the start. Make sure you have sufficient income from other sources before making commitments to take on pro bono or minimally paying clients. You may have to search for a way to make that income. I made mine by supervising associates who took my higher-paying, less dissociative clients.

Dealing with boundary violations

Write out your own feelings and discharge them in private, then write what you will say to the client so you don't explode, blame, or fail to state your concerns assertively. Confront sooner rather than later so you don't have stored-up anger and hurt. Boundary violations are inevitable. Always say "You are not in trouble." *In trouble* means a severe beating or rape that happened when they disobeyed their abusers. If boundary violations are frequent, ask the parts to turn off whatever programming is making them do this. It is important, too, that we do not invade our clients' boundaries. We can do this in many ways—offering them a ride home, touching without permission, asking intrusive questions, reading their private journal, and especially speaking with their family members. Clients may not be able to state or even know yet when their boundaries are invaded because that has been the theme of their lives so far, so it is important that we are sensitive to this possibility and reassure them that we will not be offended if they say no to anything. At the same time, there are times when our boundaries need to be extended. When I had clients who were being picked up by perpetrators right outside my office, giving a ride was helpful.

Things that interfere with therapy

Many things can interfere with the therapy process. One thing that can interfere with any client is a very busy life stage, such as the teens or young parenthood, so a person in such a stage just can't work at therapy as well as manage daily life. They might be better to postpone therapy until they have time to do the necessary work. (I have, however, had good success with some teenage survivor clients.)

But with survivors of mind control and ritual abuse, there are some specific considerations arising within or around the client:

- Your client may have distractor parts—cute playful kids, whiners and complainers, game players, itchy kids, or arguers. When you see it, name it. "Your job is to distract me, isn't it?"
- Often clients may come to therapy because they really want help. But when they arrive at your office, other parts take over and do their job of making sure no disclosures happen. When a client is being phoney (flattering you, for instance) or talking about things that don't matter, don't just go along with it. Tentatively name whatever you sense.
- Some parts of your client may have instructions to harass or burn out therapists with constant neediness. You need clear boundaries so this can't succeed.
- Clients may seem unworkable because they are still involved with (and possibly sent by) perpetrator groups. A single disclosure, or even the fact of seeing a therapist, can lead to renewed contact with abusers. For others, contact with perpetrators is ongoing no matter

what else is going on in their lives. Many survivors can still make excellent progress despite ongoing abuse and torture. It is their decision, not yours, regarding whether it is worth it for them.

- Threats to others and to you, and current actual danger, can be the basis of some survivors not working in therapy. Bring these out into the open and assess how realistic the danger is. I believe I have had clients leave me because they had been told I would be killed if they continued to see me.

- Clients can be plants, to get you to ask leading questions, invite a lawsuit, burn yourself out, or divulge information. Be careful. I had one client who was referred by her therapist mother for alleged ritual abuse involving neighbors. She did no actual work but frequently asked me if I believed her mother was part of the abuser group. I was careful to reflect the question back to her, asking whether she herself thought this. After four years, during which I'd helped her with several issues (housing, employment) not related to the alleged abuse, she politely thanked me and said four years was long enough, thank you very much.

Developing internal nurturing and independence in clients

Although many people with DID or OSDD may function well in the world, many of them are trained not to recognize, accept, and help their internal parts. With organized abuse, there is generally a rule set by the perpetrators that the front parts should have no contact with the insiders. So, a lot of internal children are abandoned. That needs to change. It begins with our caring for those child parts and other traumatized parts. Those internal parts reach out to us, but we cannot possibly meet all the needs of the very traumatized infants who should have had 24-hour loving care when the body was young. It is up to the survivor to recognize and accept those infants and provide internal caregiving.

One important thing to realize is that even these clients, even child and adolescent survivors, have had years of sadistic abuses. Healing will take years, and it cannot all depend on you, the therapist. Therapy can't last for ever. Some therapists have to relocate, some become ill, and all eventually retire. It is very important that we encourage our clients to develop internal nurturing. Their young parts do feel abandoned and grieve when therapy ends, but if they have inner adults or older children who can nurture the young ones, the sense of abandonment is less.

We begin by modeling the caring we would like to happen internally. Treat each part that emerges as the age it presents at, recognizing the developmental needs it presents. We give hugs (if we have permission) or hold the client's hand as they remember something painful. Older parts within the client observe the way we are treating the hurt parts and learn to do the same thing internally.

At the same time, we say no to demands for constant contact. We speculate out loud with adult parts about how a little child needs someone there constantly, pointing out that it's impossible now in the outside world but not in the inner world.

We can encourage the client's personality system to internalize any positive examples of nurturing and parenting they see in characters in books, movies, or TV shows, or in actual emotionally healthy adult friends. We encourage the client to designate parental nurturing parts. We might lend them parent education materials. We suggest that internal places be created where the needs of child parts can be met: a playroom, safe outdoor places, and a library of books and movies.

Plant therapists

Organized perpetrator groups have members trained as therapists. Some are actual programmers for the abuser groups and do considerable damage to the inside parts while the front parts are unaware of it. Some are just survivors who want to help others but without awareness of it continue to act according to their training to discourage remembering or awareness of parts. Survivor therapists are frequently being monitored by the perpetrator groups. It is important for a survivor to check internally with their parts and be sure that any therapist (or other professional) they go to is not harming them, reporting on them to perpetrators, or discouraging them from the things they need to do to recover fully. You as a therapist can encourage your survivor clients to check internally about responses to you in this manner, as well as exploring what their parts have to say about any previous therapists they have had. For example, did a therapist use hand signals the perpetrator group used?

Many therapists who work with survivors are themselves survivors. It's easier to work on someone else than on oneself. Do you disclose your survivor status to your client? I don't know the answer to this. Would such a disclosure be the ethical thing to do; does the survivor have a right to know? At the same time, would such a disclosure be reported by the client to their abuser group, and would it result in repercussions for you? Of course, the group may know already, as they work hard to keep track of all victims.

If you are a survivor therapist yourself, you need to check with your own insider parts to find out whether you are being monitored, whether you must report to abusers about clients, and whether you have been taught to give hand signals or other triggers to clients or discourage them from remembering their abuse. I realize these are huge and perhaps frightening tasks, but if you want to help survivors, it is important to be aware if anything is going on that could endanger you or your survivor clients. At the same time, your personal lived experience can be of immense value to help you know what is going on with such clients. Be aware, too, that a perpetrator group may send clients to use cues to trigger you and also to report about you to the group—for example, about whether you are doing any potentially effective therapy that might warrant their intervention with the client or with you.

CHAPTER 3

The life of a mind control victim

Ritual abuse and mind control by the highly organized groups is systematic and for many—though not all—victims, lifelong. The information in this chapter is very graphic. Your survivor client, who may come to you very unaware of much of what has happened to her, may have experienced most or all of what I am describing here. Much of the information here comes from Stella Katz's "A Reversed Kabbalah Trainer Speaks," pp. 91–117 in my book *Healing the Unimaginable*, Wendy Hoffman's essays in *From the Trenches*, her four memoirs, and memories shared with me by these women and other former clients of mine.

Infancy

Before the baby is born

The perpetrators administer electroshock to the pregnant mother's belly at regular intervals, beginning in the sixth month of pregnancy, sowing seeds of an attachment disorder because of the acute, distracting physical pain and shock. Their purpose is to make the mother withdraw her connection from the child. I learned this from survivors who had experienced it.

After the baby is born

The abusers give the infant physical pain right after birth, making the baby cry. If the infant accepts comforting, they will not permit the child to hold a leadership position within the perpetrator group, and may not allow it to live, as the perpetrator groups believe they would have too much difficulty trying to control the mind of a bonded child.

Hunger and dehydration are essential to prevent a nurturing bond and to lay the groundwork for dissociative splitting. No breastfeeding is allowed. The baby is kept hungry and thirsty, fed at irregular intervals and not by the mother. The group threatens that they will kill the baby unless the mother walks by and appears to ignore it. They may tell her to feed a sibling while the starving infant watches. Playing siblings against one another is standard practice.

The child is left cold and wet, sometimes with hands bound to prevent the comfort that thumb-sucking would afford. The baby, like all babies, longs to be touched and held. Someone massages the baby's feet, then inserts needles between the toes. The message is that touch leads to pain. The mother is restrained from giving comfort. When the child has been hurt, the person who is to be the child's trainer, rather than the mother, rescues the child.

Programmers teach the mother to insert fingers and then special rods to stretch the child's orifices so rapes will be manageable at an early age. If the mother won't do it, the trainer or the father does it.

The intent is to make the child form a trauma bond with the handler and/or the perpetrator group from desperation and deprivation, not love and abundance. This can create a big problem with future relationships. The baby rightfully feels no desire to want to be in this world. According to survivor Wendy Hoffman, infant feelings "form an unrelenting sack placed under the solar plexus that can follow the survivor throughout life, unless they locate these parts, rescue, and heal them" (Hoffman & Miller, 2018, p. 131).

Assessment

The trainers frighten the infant with loud noises and assess how long it takes before the child then settles. They assess the child for strength of will and dissociative ability. They use scripted traumas. They are looking for what will work best to bend this particular child or part to their wishes.

Earliest teachings

In some groups, the baby's crib has colored cloths on the sides with pockets for dolls representing the inside "people." The pockets represent the various parts' locations in the inner structures to be created in the child's mind. There are magical symbols and faces on the pockets. The child is taught how to put each foundational part in its own pocket.

Some infants are taught to pee on command and are beaten if they wet.

The first real programmed lesson is "Don't cry." There are various methods of doing this, all involving terrifying consequences of crying, in which the child may be afraid it will die. A common method is near-suffocation with a pillow. A head vise may be used. In some cases, the baby is hurt, then put into a closed box and left there until crying has stopped. No release of feelings is permitted. All feelings therefore go underground within the child.

Teaching of signals and triggers

Now the trainer teaches the infant touch triggers. Many appear to be loving touches but are reminders of pain administered while the child was semi-conscious and drugged. The child is hurt without visible marks (through electroshock or an oily substance applied to the skin). Particular touches set off particular programs (trainings). The "silence touch" is taught first: rubbing on the top of the head (at the soft spot), which will apparently calm down a survivor but actually reminds them of what will happen if they show any emotion or rebellion. I remember a survivor telling me with pride that her partner had discovered that if he touched her in this manner, she would calm right down.

The groups teach hand signals in infancy. They flutter their hands in babies' faces to sensitize them to hand motions and teach them to watch hands closely. Children learn the specific hand sequence to (for example) sit, go, lie down, fall asleep, be quiet, run, leave, enter, drop the evidence, hide something in specific places, deny, murder, shoot, kidnap, steal, poison, drop a pill in a drink, forget everything, or remember nothing. It is a kind of language.

Important words are spoken. Babies memorize words and understand them later. The basic message is "You are our possession. We own you. You will do whatever we say." Some infant parts are spoken to in occult languages.

Spinning and spinner parts

Somehow, these groups discovered quite early the use of spinning. They use it extensively and program it into personality systems. Turntables are used for babies. Stella Katz (2012, p. 104) gives a graphic description of what a baby is put through in compliance training, as every disobedient part who cries is spun at increasing speed, often vomiting many times, until the crying stops. Katz says that spinning is done at the end of a lesson (such as suicide or kill or silence) to distribute the lesson to other parts of the system. She states, "Some lessons, such as suicide or homicide, must be held by more than one alter in order for the target behavior to take place, so that one alter cannot kill the entire system, or one alter cannot kill another member of the group. Because of this kind of security measure, most people only injure themselves rather than die in their suicide attempts."

Spinning is often used at the end of an abusive episode or programming session to block the memory from being put together. When a memory is emerging, a victim becomes too dizzy to proceed.

Some groups teach a child (who becomes an internal child part) to physically spin round and round, making all other parts of the person dizzy while the one doing the spinning does not feel dizzy and keeps their balance. This spinner part is given the job of spinning internally when it is required, for example, to block a memory or to distribute sensations from a memory. If your client reports a sensation of spinning, it is an indication that a program may be running. Spinner parts can (if you ask nicely) reverse the spin in order to stop a program from working and can slowly spin something soothing and pleasant through the system to help stabilize things.

System building—first splits

At age six weeks to six months in Kabbalah-based ritual abuse groups, according to former programmer Stella Katz (2012, p. 100), the "First-born" is the first split, is not hurt again, grows up with the body, and is designated guardian of the "birth child." The Gatekeeper is the next split, keeps records of all deliberate splits, and is never hurt after his "birth," so grows up with the body. Thirteen original parts are split off, each the start of a section ("block") with a particular type of job. The splits are made by annoying sounds, needles in feet, electrodes in orifices, and other small painful shocks. The trainer watches and sees the child split, and gives each split a name, color, and symbol. The trainer keeps records in the child's "black book." Other groups' methods are similar.

Placement of original splits

In Illuminati programming, the thirteen original splits are accomplished by age six months. They are separated and placed in containers such as coffins. (This is done by placing the child in an actual coffin, which becomes internalized.) These containers are sealed and placed within the child's mind below the structure that has yet to be built internally, starting at three years old. These containers below the structure will feed the subsequent structures with feelings of hopelessness and despair. Then programmers cement the splits, color-code them, and assign them visual cues and hand signals. Some subversive programmers (like Stella Katz) deliberately and secretly leave in cracks—triggers that can unravel programming.

Trish Fotheringham, a survivor of organized abuse connected with the military (probably MK-Ultra), wrote:

> During my first weeks of life, my handlers established as much controllable dissociation as possible, as soon as possible.

Negative emotional states such as fear, helplessness, stifled anger, and loneliness, as well as positive ones such as pleasure, contentment, and safety, were isolated into separate alters. Some of these splits initially involved trauma; all were developed by giving each alter experiences that locked them steadily deeper into their emotional state ... As each base alter had enough time "out" in the body, their reality steadily began to solidify. Dissociative barriers limited their awareness to only their own pieces of my overall life. (Miller, 2012a, p. 75)

Helping inner infants

You can encourage your client to reach out to those inner infants within the mind and hold, feed, and comfort them, expressing love to them, rocking, and singing to them, keeping them warm and fed. Some survivors will know, or it may be useful to help your survivor client become aware, that their mother was forced to reject them, being a powerless victim trapped in a web of evil.

And you yourself can reach out to them, even though they cannot speak or even cry. If your eyes start to show your sorrow at what happened to them, they will be aware of it. They will feel your heart reach out to them even if you don't touch them. Sense their presence and just permit yourself to be with them, sometimes without talking.

Childhood

Growing up in the cult

The child experiences two lives simultaneously. Ordinary life has work and school, family meals, weekend outings, parties, shopping, films, sports, house cleaning, laundry, children's sports and music recitals, and homework and projects. Cult families do what normal families do in normal life. Many survivors idealize their perpetrator families.

The hidden life contains every kind of abuse: mental, physical, sexual (incest, perversion), and spiritual. Incest is enforced with parents and pets. Cult leaders mandate sexual abuse and threaten to kill kids if parents don't participate. Parents have been so abused themselves that they often, though not always, have their own perversions. Inner parts of children are sent on assignments, according to their programming. Some parents find ways to mess up a little of their children's programming.

Evaluation of child victims

Experts continue to evaluate each child to see what will motivate him or her. Will this person place their own survival first or others' survival? Which does each victim fear more: professional or public humiliation, or physical torture? Children's talents and interests are usurped for the group's purposes. Abilities may be hidden from the world and used only in cult life, where the person can be "important" and special and apparently needed. Very bright children are taught to simulate learning disabilities and can also be given actual learning disabilities.

The perpetrator groups have studied developmental stages, and their interventions at each stage are designed for brains at that stage of development. Very bright children may experience these interventions slightly earlier than regular children.

Preschool years—building the "foundation" and the inner world

The parts are designed to live in an inner world, which they experience as real. It may look like a fairy-tale world with castles, lakes, and rivers. Or it may be a group of geometric structures. Each structure has a design, such as a pyramid or a spider web. The purpose of the inner world is to give every part, and every type of part, a place where it can be found by the perpetrators when it is to be called upon for a task. Different sectors contain different kinds of insiders, some groups hidden. A section is likely to have layers, each layer having parts created at a particular age. Satanic groups create a new layer each year on the person's birthday. Within the inner world there may be control rooms with control panels, wiring, and switches, in which trained parts turn programs on and off in response to cues or dates. Different programmers over time, including those from different perpetrator groups, may create new sections and place them somewhere in the system, often hidden from the insiders created by the original trainers.

The abuser group creates the child's inner world by artificial means. For systems with geometric structures, very young children (ages three to six) are given building toys and a diagram of the structure they are to build. More artistic children may be told to draw and paint the structure. When a part succeeds in completing this task, it becomes the primary builder part. After the model of the structure is built, the child (not necessarily the same part) is told to put it inside their mind. The builder parts continue within the person's mind and may later be given or take up building tasks. Sometimes they envision themselves as adults with skills in building houses or more complex structures. Later in life, when the person is healing, builder parts can use their skills to help redesign the inner world or create better structures than the ones provided by the abuser group, ones that are more humane.

For more realistic worlds, the abusers use hypnosis, drugs, picture books, films, video games, and virtual reality to help the child visualize the places the perpetrator group wants in the child's head. They use scenery and props to make the child believe he or she is in heaven, hell, spaceships, Nazi Germany, other worlds, over the rainbow, or whatever the trainers can devise.

The original parts from whom the rest are to be split are brought forward, and each originally created part is split further to make a group of parts with the same job and type of training.

Once children get to school age, they often go to "cult camp," which is actually a week or two at a cult training center for intensive training, including some time doing actual summer camp activities. Their front parts will only remember the regular summer camp activities.

Physical methods of training

The abusers use *psychoactive drugs* to create separate biological states:

- Tranquilizers for suggestible, passive, compliant parts
- Amphetamines for rageful perpetrator parts who want to act out their anger and feel powerful
- Hallucinogens (along with suggestion) to distort perception for demon and alien parts

- Strong painkillers for parts, such as ghosts, who are not to believe they belong to the body
- Pleasure-enhancing drugs (MDMA) for use during sexual events and orgies, including when a child has to sexually abuse others
- Antipsychotics for front parts to block awareness of other inside people.

The groups use all known methods of *torture* on children. They have a portable shock helmet that delivers electric shock to specific brain areas and a special chair that delivers electric shocks as well as drugs, spinning, and the sensation of flight. Pain in particular spots on the body may be used to create parts who "live" there. Electroshock is important in sealing off training sessions for the various programs.

Terror is basic. There are threats to the child's life with guns, whips, waterboarding, and suffocation to the point of unconsciousness. After witnessing both real and simulated murders, the child victim believes that noncompliance will result in death.

Emotional methods of training

Deprivation is used extensively. There is sensory deprivation. The child victim is locked in a deprivation room, thrown into a pit, put in a crawl space. Cages and chains are used extensively.

Overwhelm is also used. Noise is used for sensory overload, combined with hallucinogens to program children to be "crazy." As previously mentioned, spinning is used from infancy to overwhelm children and teach children they have no control over their own bodies.

Shame is basic. The child is put in double binds and given forced choices such as "You kill this animal, or we kill this child," followed by the message that the child is evil because it is a killer. There is a lot of deliberate shaming, humiliation, and belittlement. In ritually abusive groups, there is simulation of heaven and hell, with rejection by "God" and "Jesus" and apparent acceptance by "Satan" and "Lucifer," with the invitation to perpetrate instead of being harmed. (See Chapter 9.)

If you let awareness of all this sink in, you will have more compassion for your clients who have gone through this, and that compassion will reach their hidden parts.

Deception in training

All the training and programming of victims relies heavily on deception. There is a difference between what is really happening and what the perpetrators tell the child is happening. Along with the torture and threats, the abusers use many deceptions and illusions. When an adult survivor remembers these events, they may be confused by the deceptions.

Hypnosis is combined with drugs and stage magic to confuse victims. Trish Fotheringham's account ("Mind Control as I Experienced It," 2012a, pp. 74–85) lists "theatrics, illusion, sets, sounds, smells, costumes, makeup, elaborate role-plays." The abusers place cameras and microphones in places where they are not present, then tell the victim (with examples) that they know everything the victim says and does. Victims in their sixties and older report the use of picture cards, photographs, mirrors, storybooks, nursery rhymes, and fairy tales. Victims in their forties and fifties remember films. Younger victims remember virtual reality, holograms, and computer-generated images. As mentioned in Chapter 2, they remember simulated surgeries to implant supposed bombs, a black heart, Satan's brain, tracking devices, or an animal that will eat the victim's internal organs if they talk about the abuse. For more about deception, see my 2019 presentation for the Survivorship conference: https://ritualabuse.us/smart-conference/2019-conference/deception-by-organized-abuser-groups-helping-your-front-people-and-your-insiders-recognize-the-lies-and-tricks-which-keep-you-enslaved-by-alison-miller/.

Indoctrination

Beliefs are hammered into victims over and over through religious ceremonies, military drills, songs and chants and rhymes, rewards, and punishments. The primary message is the superiority of the perpetrator group: "We have superior knowledge and wisdom. We serve the correct deity in the correct way. Our way of life is the only right way, and our leader or deity deserves obedience and loyalty. You can trust our group because we are your family, the only ones who care about you. We do these things [abuses] for your own good, to train you and make you strong.

We are going to make the world a better place." Any indication of disbelief in a victim leads to severe punishment, so parts who believe these statements split off, even though the core of the person knows these are lies.

Obedience and loyalty

Obedience is expected to be instant. "You belong to us [a slave, though this word is not always used]. You are good if you obey us and bad if you disobey." Just as in many regular families, obedience is highly valued, and obedient children are proof of excellent parenting; so it is within these multigenerational groups, only more so. There is punishment for minor infractions. There are rewards for obedience and doing one's job. The abuser groups give such rewards as pleasurable drugs (opiates), pleasurable sex (such as gentle touch or orgasm without pain), getting to abuse another child instead of being abused, stripes on the military uniform (for "soldier" parts), and rings (for promotions).

Child victims (who become child parts of your adult client) are told they are robots, computers, sex machines, killing machines, anything other than human beings. They are told, "You were created only to do the job assigned to you. You will have no purpose and will not exist if you don't do it." Those parts believe they will cease to exist if they don't do their jobs for the perpetrators.

Many groups train children as soldiers. Everyone in "developed" countries was shocked when information came out about child soldiers in African terror groups. The same thing is happening in a hidden way in developed countries and has been for generations. Abusers dress children in uniforms, put them through military exercises, show them movies of soldiers marching or fighting, give promotions, and talk about pride in the cause. The "commanders" punish children who cry, vomit, show fear or sadness, or show compassion for others being hurt. For example, they say: "You are a soldier whose duty is to obey without thinking, never think for yourself. If you obey, you will rise to be a general (or another high rank). If you fight back, you are a traitor and will be punished." There are court-martials for disobedient soldier parts.

Troops of children are marched with guns and told to shoot enemy troops. They shoot in unison, and the enemy troops (also children) fall down, apparently lifeless. When you hear this from a client, ask whether any other part of that client has memories of being told to march and then to fall down and keep still when the enemies' guns went off. The answer is likely to be yes. Because of dissociation, the parts who "killed" and the parts who "were killed" were unaware of one another.

The group leaders call a disloyal group member (initially a child) a traitor, tell the children that traitors deserve rape and/or torture and/or death, and demonstrate this punishment. The authorities remind the victim that "We can kill you or take you away at any time, and no one can stop us because we are all-powerful." If this doesn't work to get loyalty and obedience, the group raises the ante: "If you are disloyal, someone you love, or another vulnerable child, will be killed or punished instead of you." Large gatherings are staged, in which all the children of group members observe the ritual murder (real or staged) of someone who is said to be a traitor. Leaders may make children hold the knife and stab the body.

The parts who are designed to have internal authority within the personality system are told they must make the other parts obey, and they (the internal leaders) will be punished if those under their authority disobey the perpetrators. The groups put designated internal leaders through ceremonies in which they make vows and solemn promises to be loyal and obedient. Sometimes they sign in blood.

Meanwhile, the front parts of the child, the ones who live an ordinary life, know nothing about this.

Lies they tell

In *From the Trenches*, I wrote an essay entitled "Fifty Lies They May Have Told You" (Hoffman & Miller, 2018, pp. 53–84). Each specific lie has a specific purpose. Lies are backed up by trickery (fake stage magic, illusions, and drugs). My list of fifty lies has the lie, the truth, why the perpetrators tell this lie, how they make their victims believe it, and what to do about it. If your client wants to read this essay, I suggest they first write down statements abusers made that they suspect may be lies, but they aren't sure. Then they can see whether the lies they suspect are on the list. There are lies about the reality of the abuse, about the abusers' power and character, about obedience and disobedience, about the necessity of keeping in contact with the abusers, about what will happen if the victim tells someone about the abuse, about life and death and reality, and about what or who the victim is.

The lies are, of course, combined with "evidence" of their truth. The secret lies told to children are reinforced by the public lies (disinformation) spread throughout society. The trick to making disinformation believable is to include plenty of correct information that is already known, so the speaker or writer is not revealing anything new. Learning critical thinking is an important part of recovery for victims of these abuses.

Child victims hear many of the group's lies constantly from family members. Parts are trained to remind other parts, especially the front parts, of the lies.

The BIG LIE

To control someone when they aren't in your presence, you must make them believe such things as: you always know where they are, you know what they are doing and thinking, you have the power to kill them or their loved ones at any time without getting caught, and you are the only ones who can keep them safe.

The BIG LIE of these abusers, which they tell their child victims, is: "We know everything and are all-powerful. We have magical [or technological] ways of knowing what you think and do and say." This lie is one important way of preventing victims from telling what has happened and is happening to them and also puts pressure on all parts to do their jobs.

There are many versions of this. The walls have ears (simulated.) God/Lucifer/Satan (who is omnipotent, omniscient, and omnipresent) is always watching you. You see his eyes (a memory of eyes on the wall). Mothers have eyes in the back of their heads. We (the almighty perpetrator group) live in the shadows or in the walls wherever you go. The crows/squirrels/spiders (insert the most common animal in the victim's locality) report to us. Your stuffed animals report to us. A microchip or device implanted in your body tells us where you are and what you are thinking and saying. A bomb in your body will go off if you are disloyal.

All these things are simulated in childhood, using hidden microphones, one-way mirrors, fake surgeries, and other deceptions. The gist of it, whatever lie they use, is that it is impossible to hide anything from the perpetrator group, so victims must tell the group everything.

Huh? Why would the group need victims to tell them things if they already know those things? Just plain logic defeats this lie if you think about it. Help your client think about it, as your client's reporter parts are required to tell a designated member of the abuser group about any disloyalty.

One version of the BIG LIE that may be largely true is "Everyone you know is linked to us and will report to us." Victims' friends are for the most part assigned by the perpetrator group, and victims are made to report on one another. There is programming to tell only the truth to people who give the signal that indicates they are sent by the group and never to tell the truth to outsiders. Another possibility of a truth here is that there may well be recording going on—by the victim's cellphone. Are your clients bringing those phones into therapy sessions? They may be recording your sessions.

The orchestrated sacrifice of a friend

(See Stella Katz's personal essay in *Healing the Unimaginable*, 2012, p. 211, and Wendy Hoffman's personal account in *The Enslaved Queen*, 2014, pp. 85–96.)

I have heard this from enough survivors to believe it is a common practice. At around age six, the child is given a friend, usually another child, carefully chosen from the sacrificial victims bred for this purpose, and not known to the outside world. The victim child, who is not designed to be sacrificed, has never been permitted a friend before, and has known no love or even kindness, so this is a very special relationship. It is hard for normal people to imagine the hunger these children have for love and connection. The relationship lasts about a year, and then the child who has tasted love is forced to participate in the murder of his or her friend. The mind control message is that love is not allowed, that the cult leaders will murder any person or animal you love.

After that, if anyone the child knows becomes ill or injured or dies, the child is told it is his or her fault. The important message is, "Don't love anyone, or that person will be killed." This has devastating, lifelong effects for the victim.

However, this can backfire, as the victim now knows what love is, knows that they can be loved by someone who is capable of love, and has hope it may happen again, as well as fear for anyone who may love them. Some victims have told me that the deceased special friend has remained with the victim and shielded him or her from the full impact of the torture. The abusers may try to teach the victim to displace the love felt for the sacrificed friend to a target person designated to be the child's friend or lover (and often handler). But this first love may be too strong for this displacement to work completely.

Forced perpetration

Occult groups force children to participate in torture, rape, animal sacrifice, and real and simulated murders. Even if the murder is a simulation, the child does not know it. Training begins with forcing the child to kill a pet with which they have been allowed to bond. The trainer's hand is over the child's hand, then the child is blamed for the death and told he or she is evil. The message to the child is "Kill or be killed." And subsequently, "You are a murderer, and no good person will ever want to know you." (See Chapter 9 for more details.)

False and cover memories

Even though there is strong "don't tell" programming, the perpetrator groups are always aware of the danger of memories of their abuses leaking out and the survivor telling someone who might believe them. So, they set up false memories. One such memory is the murder of a person the child knows in the "real" world, such as at school. The child attends a ritual or other event in which that person is apparently murdered. The child is encouraged to report this to the police. The police investigate and find the person alive and well. I have had more than one survivor tell me about this. The memory of the faked murder is designed to come up if the victim is beginning to remember real crimes. Another such memory is the standard alien abduction, complete with spaceship and "aliens" doing things to the child's body with instruments. Meanwhile, cover memories cover the time periods when horrible things happened. For example, "Cult camp" includes training by perpetrator groups, and films or brief experiences of actual camp serve as cover memories. A client of mine was regularly abducted while walking along the railway tracks from town to the home in which she was hiding; a part of her was trained to replace the memories of the abductions with memories of actually walking along those tracks safely.

Horrendous sexual training and abuse

Where do the perpetrator groups get the funding for all the things they do? Much of it comes from selling children's bodies or images of child sexual abuse. Some perpetrator groups exist primarily for this purpose, while others get funded this way but have different overall goals. For example, military groups make use of sexually skilled seducers and spies, and political groups as well as traditional organized crime groups use their victims for blackmail purposes.

Children are taught to have sexual feelings toward any person the trainer points to. These sexual programs are sometimes turned on accidentally and lead to unfortunate outcomes. If your client tries to seduce you, they are probably acting on such programming.

Children are trained very early to be used sexually and to please adults with perverse sexual appetites. Children are forced to engage in mixed pain and pleasure and extreme sexual perpetration with one another, adults, dead bodies, and animals. They are trained by being masturbated while watching filmed then actual violence. Some sexual trainings take place in electroshock chairs, where children are masturbated and then electroshocked on their genitals and nipples to couple their premature sexual feelings with physical pain. They are masturbated before or while being tortured or being placed next to dead bodies.

Pain holder parts are brought out simultaneously with the masochist and perpetrator parts so the ones who feel the pleasure don't feel the pain their bodies experience or inflict.

Frequently victims are trained so that they cannot experience orgasm unless in a violent situation, either hurting someone or being hurt by someone. Assassins and those who kill in ceremonies are trained to experience orgasm when someone is killed. Drugs are used to enhance both sexuality and anger. Pairing intense sexual pleasure with violence can lead to the creation of child parts who are incapable of empathy and associate sexual pleasure only with violence or near-death. Pedophilic and violent sexual offenders should be routinely assessed for dissociative disorders.

One very sad thing about this is that the perpetrator groups may turn some of their victims into their customers for the material they produce. When we look at the changes in society over recent years, with violent and extreme and drugged sex becoming normalized, we may wonder whether the perpetrator groups have created this change.

It is possible to remove urges for harmful sexual behavior such as pedophilia by processing memories that caused the split between pain or empathy parts and parts who experience orgasm. For an example, see Meredith Sharman's account "My Sexual Healing Process" in *Becoming Yourself* (Miller, 2014, pp. 265–271) and chapter 14, "Treating Programmed Pedophilia," pp. 225–234 of *Healing the Unimaginable* (Miller, 2012a).

A breeder, primarily in adolescence, has the job of giving birth to infants for sacrifice or sale. She may have an unregistered child who is used for torture training and is kept until a scheduled date of sacrifice. These are very hard memories for survivors to deal with.

Tasks in sexual recovery

Reconnecting sexuality with love and caring is a major task and can only be attempted after other recovery work. Most survivors become divorced from their bodies. Celibacy may be preferable in the meantime. It is the survivor's choice whether they want full sexual healing. Most survivors find these memories too painful to approach. One of my clients used to ask me regularly to promise her that she would never have to have sex again. I supported her in this.

Survivors with loving partners sometimes want to heal their sexuality for the sake of their partners, or to regain their full being. First steps include: learning to accept the body they have, getting in touch with their body and their senses in a more general sense, figuring out their sexual orientation, dealing with sexual acting out, figuring out their sexual values, and partner communication. Figuring out the person's sexual orientation can be difficult. One male survivor despised two of his parts who kept urging him to have sex with men, though his front parts were heterosexual. It turned out that as a boy he had been forced to have sex with men in order to obtain the reward of loving touch from a woman, and that is what these parts wanted.

Once a survivor's personality system is cooperative and decides to work towards sexual recovery, here are some internal tasks that a survivor needs to accomplish: accessing their history of sexual victimization, facing up to their history of sexual perpetration, having victim parts share their feelings with perpetrator parts, working through the sexual training memories, and dealing with their history of "breeder" pregnancies for those who have a female body. Men and boys need to deal with having been used to impregnate breeders or to punish disobedient victims through rape. Then external tasks: trying solo sex, noticing and permitting unusual arousing thoughts or fantasies without acting on them in inappropriate ways. Then engaging in sex with a kind, patient, and non-threatening partner. Learning not to allow themselves to be used. Giving sexual parts permission to love their sexual partner, and finally, allowing themselves sexual enjoyment with this partner. That is quite a list. I developed it from Meredith Sharman's account of how she did it.

Anger and love displacement training

Programmers manipulate anger in children, starting almost at birth. They deliberately frustrate and enrage infants by taking away love, bottles, pacifiers, soft objects to cuddle, sometimes giving them to a sibling or another child. They isolate the anger into certain parts of the child and train those parts. By the time their victims are toddlers, they are training them to kill. At four to six years old, kids are taught to direct their anger (which is really at the perpetrators) toward the group's enemies, including anyone who tries to help the child victims escape. Wendy Hoffman wrote about this in in her essay "Anger Displacement Training," in *From the Trenches* (Hoffman & Miller, 2018, pp. 138–141). The parts of a survivor trained to aim the survivor's anger at specific people may well be called on to aim it at you, if the client is making progress with your therapy.

Besides anger displacement training, there is also love displacement training. The love the child may genuinely feel for someone, such as the friend who was sacrificed, is to be displaced onto whoever the perpetrators want the child to love: for example, the person the group wants the person to marry, a cult-involved therapist, or a handler.

Events specific to Satanic and Luciferian ritual abuse

Satanism and Luciferianism are genuine religions. Like any religion, they have rituals and traditions, and despite what the Satanic Temple people might tell you, they have very unpleasant rituals. Rituals are conducted on both Christian and pagan holidays. Not all ritual abuse stars Satan or Lucifer. There is ritual abuse in the name of Christ. "The special child's spiritual training" (pp. 57–66 of *Healing the Unimaginable*) is a survivor's accounts of "Christian" (Freemason) and Luciferian ritual abuse in the same church by the same people in different costumes.

Important rituals often involve animal and human sacrifice. Street people and unregistered children are usually the victims.

In reversed Kabbalah training with Hebrew letters and/or tarot cards, the child walks pathways, outdoors or in a cult training center, with different doors leading to different events, most of them painful, all designed to teach something. The groups simulate demons in training centers by puppets and film. They put costumes on children and tell them they are demons.

There is simulation of the afterlife, including heaven and hell, with religious figures, God and Jesus, and sometimes pagan gods or gods of ancient religions. (See Chapter 9.)

There are milestone events for every child:

Satanic baptism is a painful rape of a child aged twelve to eighteen months by a man in a devil suit during a ritual.

Satanic rebirth is a ritual involving sewing a child aged around six inside the body of a beast, from which a strong part of the child fights its way out and is welcomed as a leader of the child's personality system.

Marriage to Satan is the child's official loss of virginity in a ritual at around age nine, although the child has experienced many rapes prior to this. In this ritual, the child is dressed up beautifully as a bride, then is raped by her "husband," the man (cult leader) in the devil suit.

A teenage girl's firstborn male child is considered "*Satan's child*" and is sacrificed, usually by the girl herself, who is forced to do it. The part of her who conducts the sacrifice may or may not know she gave birth to the baby, and if she knows, she may want this baby to die rather than have a life like her own.

The "angel" of suicide

One important suicide program is "the welcoming angel." Images of this angel and persons dressed as this angel lead the way into a supposed paradise of comfort and peace. The angel looks beautiful, like a Renaissance painting. In the crib, before the infant knows speech, handlers show images of the angel as they stroke, soothe, drug, and feed the famished baby. They use technical equipment to project the fake angel's picture around and across the room, as if it were flying. Programmers torture the child, then drug the unfortunate infant and show the image of the angel, which becomes associated with relief. See Wendy Hoffman's essay about this angel in *From the Trenches* (Hoffman & Miller, 2018, pp. 167–169).

In reversed Kabbalah cult training centers, after much torture and terror, in the last room at the end of each pathway there may be a woman dressed up as the angel who drugs the child and soothes her into sleep. Parts are taught to try to commit suicide when they see the image of the angel, believing they will be welcomed into the presence of the soothing angel.

Later, perpetrators can command this suicide through a signal that elicits the internal image of the angel.

Adulthood

Arranged adult lives

Some people are only of use to their perpetrator groups when they are children and can be used for sexual exploitation. They have no value to the perpetrators in adulthood. Some are not easily trainable. If they are not seen as a threat to the group's security, these people have their systems "closed down" in adolescence and are not used in adulthood, although some of these have training to return for a checkup at certain ages. It is important to determine whether your client is closed down or is someone who will be expected to remain part of the perpetrator group for life. In any case, even those who are closed down or discarded usually have programming to report to perpetrators if they start to disclose secrets of the perpetrator group (see Chapter 7). In some cases, the perpetrator group has disbanded or died out.

What I am saying in this section applies to the many victims who have not been thoroughly closed down and abandoned by their perpetrator groups. The perpetrator group arranges these victims' lives, even when victims believe they have made their own choices. The group has assessed the victims' interests and abilities, and places them in careers that will benefit the group.

Most cult marriages are prearranged. The spouse may be a group member or a handler, or may just be someone with their own childhood trauma who can be easily intimidated by the perpetrators and trained to keep the victim in line. Only some parts of the victims are aware of this. The group chooses victims' living locations, either so that the group can access them or so that the group can exile them when they are no longer of use. There are cult neighborhoods, cult retirement communities, cult monitoring communities where disloyal victims are sent to live and be watched closely, and cult-owned properties around graveyards where rituals are conducted and dead bodies are available.

In some cases, front parts are trained to remain loyally with one religious group that has enough members of the perpetrator group in its leadership to control victims throughout life. Perpetrator group leaders give hand signals from the pulpit while spouting Christian beliefs.

Survivors are sent to cult-involved therapists, sometimes called plants. Survivor therapists are sent cult-involved clients to give signals and warnings. Cults provide training for their therapists to close down survivors' memories. Some cult-involved therapists are sophisticated programmers, and victims of high value to the perpetrators are sent to these therapists.

If a victim starts to rebel or to work on their memories, the perpetrators may make sure that the victim has a child or a pet to protect to motivate the victim to be compliant. Many people will give in to perpetrators to save others, especially those they love, from the same fate.

Spies, knowing and unknowing

Victims' friends tend to be other victims, even when neither party is aware of it. All victims have parts taught to report on other victims. The perpetrators decide who victims' friends will be, choosing from among their members people who fit a certain type that the victim will find attractive. Conferences, websites, and online discussion groups for survivors are all infiltrated by programmers and spies and slaves who give triggers for programmers. Some resources for survivors are actually run by perpetrator groups. They give superficial help while monitoring survivors and making sure no one gets free. If a new person appears in a survivor's life, that person may have been sent by the perpetrator group as a handler or a spy.

Handlers (minders)

A victim who has not been closed down and let go is likely to have a handler (some groups use the term "minder" for a lower-level handler) until they escape or die. A handler makes sure the victim follows all commands, that their programs remain intact, that they make no moves toward breaking free. Reporting parts of the victim, usually young child parts, make sure the handlers know what is going on, compulsively telling everything that is happening to them. The same handler can monitor many people's lives. Handlers can be parents, siblings, spouses, lovers, relatives, children, friends, therapists—or clients. Handlers are demoted and punished if their victims break free. Although there is programming only to tell the truth to handlers, a recovering victim may be able to defeat that programming and then lie to their handler rather than reporting the truth about what they are thinking and feeling and planning.

This is each victim's life trajectory, unless the victim makes an enormous effort to break free. It is horrifying and sad. But we can help the victims we treat to break free and regain their true selves and their autonomy. Those who were used only in childhood and are no longer of value to the perpetrators may not be as closely monitored and may find the healing process easier.

Becoming "conscious" perpetrators

A "conscious" member of the perpetrator group is fully identified with the goals of the group, rewarded with status, power, and freedom from being tortured. The group gives people designated for leadership due to genetics or abilities the opportunity to become "conscious" perpetrators when they reach a certain age, usually thirty-three or thirty-nine. The opportunity to "go conscious" is presented to candidates, who must agree to it. Some who were designated for leadership may refuse. Even Satanists and Luciferians have rules about agreements being important.

In a "conscious" person, the cult-identified parts of the person have integrated with the front people, keeping the hidden tortured and rebellious child parts buried deep inside, never to emerge. Conscious members are aware of what they are triggering and why. They may become programmers or "matriarchs" (women who keep other members in childlike dependency) or have other responsibilities that contribute to the agenda of the perpetrator group. They often have high positions in society.

The groups' activities in the wider world

Perpetrator groups collaborate and teach one another techniques of torturing children, splitting the infant mind, and training mind-controlled victims. This is psychologically sophisticated organized crime, which runs in families. There is a high level of national and international organization of these groups. They collaborate on training centers.

Mind control of populations

These abuser groups have, I believe, been experimenting with mind control of entire populations. The basic principles are the same, whether in mind control of a single human brain or mind control of a population. Create a traumatic event (or use one that has happened), create a split between parts reacting to the event, train those parts how to respond, create or select strong autocratic leaders who will control those below them, control communications (in society, this means the media) so that underlings only know what they are told to "know." We see the results of this population mind control in many societies today. Below are some specific training methods that abuser groups have used to contribute to societal mind control.

Politicians' use of victims

High-level perpetrator groups make money from sexual abuse but have political goals, wanting to have their loyal members in power. The major cult groups (such as Illuminati and Nazis) select from among their trainees suitable persons who are scheduled to be in political power eventually. Victims are trained to service these people as sexual slaves, memorizers, and messengers. Memorizer parts of such victims are taught to use their brains as a camera or tape recorder, recording words and documents. Messenger parts deliver elite drugs and/or messages and instructions in writing. Other parts are trained to assassinate politicians. The perpetrator groups work hard to disguise the identities of publicly well-known perpetrator group members, doing special identity confusion training for victims after encounters with such people.

Gang wars and the bandwagon

The groups train victims to join an angry cause. They must do or say whatever they are told to do or say by the group's leader. The training is to be part of a "gang" and "get on the bandwagon" when given the correct cue. Trainers say, "You will always follow your leader. You will always join your team. You will always protest when they protest injustice." Injustice is the key false-word. "You express the anger while your team leader is quiet. Sometimes you will not know who your team leader is. You are the voice for justice." We have seen examples of the results of this training in recent public events. See Wendy Hoffman's essay "Gang wars and the bandwagon" in *From the Trenches* (Hoffman & Miller, 2018, pp. 145–148.)

Assassin training

Little girls are trained to seduce, perform lap dances, drop pills in victims' drinks, and escape as the victims become drowsy, sick, or die. They are also trained to pull the triggers of guns. These child parts exist within adult survivors.

Kids who will become assassins are trained to aim at archery and shooting ranges. For the "big job", they are trained to arrive at the destination, switch to the next inner part in a sequence of trained parts, position themselves, switch, aim, switch, watch for a handler's signal, switch, practice aim and reposition, switch, obey a signal, switch, shoot, and finally switch into a part who knows nothing about what just happened. The same part does not perform the whole act. A sequence of seven to ten parts, isolated from the rest of the brain, are trained with a metronome, to hypnotize them, and a stick pounding, to accelerate the switches from one brain part to the next. A sequence of songs in the head can be used. Words, hand and foot signals, icons, or sounds open the program. Assassins have suicide pills. Some are trained to stay put and be captured, some to run and be captured, some to escape. They are kept as fringe citizens. When a group assassinates a public figure, other killers shooting from other directions disappear undetected. The expendable assassin is discovered with a gun. There are perpetrator group members among the investigators. (See Hoffman's essay "How to make an assassin" in *From the Trenches*, pp. 142–144.)

CHAPTER 4

Engineered personality systems

The programmers working for these organized perpetrator groups engineer the personality systems of their victims, placing parts in specific locations in what the victim describes as an inner world and assigning them all roles that benefit the perpetrator group. Although there may be hundreds or even thousands of parts, it is still one person, one brain: one very badly hurt person, and a brain that had to adapt to living with hidden torture and an unknowing and uncaring outside world.

Trainers instruct parts to engage in their trained behaviors in response to specific conditioned stimuli. We therapists can come to understand the kinds of training programs and the jobs parts have been assigned. We can help the parts work together to resolve the trauma and create a cooperative and gradually integrating personality system.

Sections within the brain

Early in the child victim's life, the perpetrator group creates the different sections of inner people. The major sections may belong to different perpetrator groups who have different ideas and purposes. Each section begins with one insider part, from whom the rest of the parts of a particular type are split. By "insider", I mean a part who is not permitted to come out into the body in ordinary life but comes out in response to a command from the perpetrator group.

The trainers give each initial insider a set of cues, each of which will bring him or her out to do his or her job. A cue may be visual, like a playing card or a picture or a raised eyebrow, or auditory, like a song hummed or a series of knocks or the part's assigned name, or tactile, like a particular touch.

Stella Katz's essay "A Reversed Kabbalah Trainer Speaks," in *Healing the Unimaginable* (Miller, 2012a, pp. 91–117), describes thirteen foundational blocks of parts made by such groups. Over the years, the personality system is developed, like a tree with branches, until there are many parts of each type, all split (through torture) from the first part of that type. Sections may be assigned specific colors to identify them. Most of the "people," even if they have names, are not very substantial but may just have one skill or obey one order. When a particular skill combination is needed for a task, the cues for each skill needed are shown, resulting in a temporary person who has that combination of abilities or traits. The temporary part may have a hyphenated name like Mary-Louise because it combines Mary and Louise.

Insiders' jobs

Most insiders have specialized "jobs" in which they have been trained. Some jobs are always to be done; other jobs are to be done in response to certain types of events in the inner or outer world. Some jobs involve action in the outside world, such as reporting to family members about therapy, opening doors in response to a specific knock, coming when called by a hand signal, memorizing and conveying messages, sexual slavery, assassination, ritual sacrifice, or speaking Satanic languages in rituals. Other jobs are done in the inside world, such as keeping records of training events, watching the person's behavior in order to report any disloyalty, distributing programs, giving orders, punishing non-compliant parts, turning programs on or off, frightening child parts, and reactivating programs. Most insiders engage in "forced labor," doing jobs out of fear for themselves or fear of others being killed or tortured.

All insiders with jobs have several (often thirteen) backups, others who will take over their jobs if an original insider decides not to do its job. For this reason, it is important to ask the backups to listen and respond when you negotiate with any part around quitting its job (and possibly taking on a new role that will benefit the person instead of the perpetrator group).

Some backups are parts who had the same job at an earlier age. Others are created with "duplicate programming," which takes a part newly trained and makes the system create many duplicates of that part. I have heard of this being done by placing a young child inside a structure such as a ball that has mirrors all around the inside of it, then spinning that structure while administering many small pains to the child. The "duplicates" created in this way are rather insubstantial copies of the original part, but have the same job as the original part, usually something regarding obedience or loyalty to the perpetrator group.

In this book, I have described the different kinds of programs I have seen in survivors. The way I learned about these was when they were triggered in my clients. Sometimes a client's disobedience to basic rules triggered a program. Sometimes an order from the local perpetrator group or a communication from family members elsewhere was the trigger. In either case, a part began to do its job, and through communication with the system about that job, the program was revealed to me. You can do the same thing. There are a variety of ways in which a particular lesson is taught in the perpetrator groups, and you can discover the jobs of various parts of your client, and the training that gave them these jobs, by noticing when they are triggered to do those jobs.

Basic programming for all parts

No matter what the part's location, age, or specific job, it has this basic programming:

1. Be loyal and obedient to the perpetrator group
2. Don't talk to any outsider about the abuse or the abusers
3. Don't love anyone (or they will die, or your energy will harm them)
4. Accept only the "friends" or spouses or family members the group sends you
5. Don't trust any outsider.

Appearing normal: the front

Front people

Front people are the parts of the person who deal primarily with every-day life in the known and relatively safe world. There may be more than one front part, but as they change place seamlessly, other people may not notice. Front parts are trained not to be aware of or remember the abuse, even if it is ongoing. Several front people may share the job, and the person's memory or behavior depends on which ones are present at the time. Often the front person is a "shell" that contains different com-binations of parts at different times. Or it may be a "stage" upon which different groups of players act out their roles.

Survivors usually have a series of front people as they age. When one is traumatized or finds the job too stressful, that part may be replaced by a new front part. Different ones have different skills. They seem to share recent memory, but not memory of trauma. There is usually a strong bar-rier against the front people knowing anything about the other inside parts or communicating with them. Within the inner world, parts may see a huge crevasse or a wall of fire between the front and the rest of the system. Perpetrators strictly forbid communication through the barrier.

The front part (known to some therapists as the "apparently normal personality" (ANP)) of a person who is multiple was formerly known as the "host," which gave the inaccurate impression that this part is some-how more real than the other parts, who are more like guests, welcome or unwelcome. The front person of a multiple often feels as if they are somehow unreal (depersonalization). They may feel as if the world is unreal, or they are in the wrong time or place (derealization). They are likely to hear voices in their head, often critical or giving orders or com-menting on their life and behavior. They may or may not realize that there are other parts within the brain.

Programming for front people

Front people are trained, just as other parts are. Their specific rules or tasks are:

1. Appear normal
2. Keep emotions under control

3. Don't hear voices
4. Don't communicate internally
5. Don't remember the abuse.

Do you work with the front person?

There are therapists who believe you should only work with the front person (part), as if that part is more real than the others. I disagree strongly. Whether you work with the front person at all (other than greeting them at the door) depends on the functionality of the front person. If a front person has years of high functioning, you may be able to work with the other parts through that front person, and the inner parts may respect that front part, who brings much strength and experience. But in many cases, if not most, the front person is only a shell, so it's wiser not to bother trying to work with or through them, as they do not have the information that the survivor needs to resolve their trauma and dissociation. You should keep in touch with the front person in order to know about their everyday life, work, and health. But the bulk of the work needs to be with the insiders. Front people and insider parts often hate one another. You need to do mediation, explaining to each what the other's purpose is and why they are the way they are. Front people are specialized for handling day-to-day life and have little or no awareness of the trauma history. In many cases, that awareness would traumatize them and interfere with their functioning. Insiders hide the pain, the anger, the overwhelming knowledge, and the strong emotions.

Moderators and modulators

I have heard of these parts only from survivors who told me about them, and it is possible that only victims who are supposed to hold high office within the perpetrator groups have these parts. They operate behind the front people in everyday life (including therapy sessions) to smooth things out. A moderator I met had the job of making the person's speech sound like an adult of the age she was, regardless of the age of the part who was communicating, so that a listener would not recognize the presence of a child part. A modulator I met smoothed things out in other ways, making sure that communications to other people were all reviewed and made acceptable to the listener, while not revealing protected or sensitive information.

Denial programming

Denial is programmed into survivors, especially the front people, and is very tempting for the victim. Not knowing gives a survivor an illusion of a happy childhood and a loving family. Families involved in perpetrator groups offer survivors some semblance of family life in exchange for not remembering and not telling. We are tempted to deny the reality, along with our clients. Denial must be overcome in order to grieve. This is true for our clients and also for us.

All front people have denial programming or training. Specific types of denial programs include:

- Forget and don't remember any of the abuse (separate programs)
- There must be no communication with inside parts, so don't hear their voices
- Only front people are to come out into the present-day world
- Don't believe your own memories.

This is the state of a survivor client when they first come to see you. They may or may not have remembered some of the things that happened to them. But denial programming is very active. Moderator and/or modulator parts may be making any part who speaks sound like an adult, if the client has such parts. Behind the front people you see, other parts are actively assessing you, whether you are a perpetrator, whether you can stand the horror, and whether there is a chance you could help them.

Distractors and confusers

These may be among the kinds of parts you meet early in therapy. They may disrupt therapy sessions by being cute, mute, or itchy, going to sleep, or changing the subject. Cute little kids will suddenly pop out and engage you in childish conversation to distract you from the important work. Mute parts will be put out and unable to speak. Itching is both a distraction and a reminder; each itch carries a message to the survivor.

The distractors and confusers have the job of diverting the survivor's attention to other things, especially current events in their everyday lives, when you are getting close to important information. Some can cause the client to forget what just happened or what was just remembered. There may be "chameleon" parts who pretend to be other specific parts whom you know.

Programs you see in the therapy room

Since disclosures to a therapist are strictly forbidden, various parts start to do their specific jobs as soon as your survivor client comes to see you. Some internal parts may start to remember that they have perpetrated. And that all therapists are abusers. And that if you look at a therapist, that therapist will rape you. If the front people have remembered abuse, some other parts may be making them remember impossible apparent memories. Internal leaders may be telling other parts to make sure to answer the therapist's questions with lies. Some parts remind others that the abusers can hear everything they hear and perhaps even think. Some parts may make others see their handler in the therapy room. Some parts may want to run, and others have training to kill or harm anyone who is kind to them. A survivor must overcome all this just to make a little progress. You can be sure that it takes a great deal of courage for your client even to make an appointment, let alone talk to you about their life.

Programs and jobs of parts

Internal hierarchies

In many (but not all) mind-controlled or cult personality systems, parts are set up in one or more hierarchies. Hierarchies often result from progressive splits with a new layer built each year from age three to about thirteen (e.g., Satan 1, Satan 2, Satan ... 9). Each layer will have one of each important type (job category), split from the previous one. The last-made layer is placed in charge of the person's behavior, and all parts must obey the ones above them. The bosses at various levels issue threats to those under them who disobey the rules. The enforcers administer punishments for disobedience, such as flashbacks, self-harm, or pain (from memories). A survivor may have different hierarchies with different bosses created by different perpetrator groups that are all under the same Satanic or organized abuse umbrella. These often clash, as in civil wars. I shall discuss hierarchies in more detail in Chapter 6.

The internal resistance

A tortured child is a person with some degree of free will, and when a child is being tortured, parts may split off that are not under the control of the abuser group, even though most parts do what they have been told to do in order to make the pain stop, or to save their life, or to save others' lives. There are parts that the abuser group can't control.

Garbage (rubbish) kids

During a training episode, especially one designed to make a child do harm, many parts may be split off, one after another, each one refusing to obey, until the person eventually recognizes that resistance is futile and just gives up and allows a non-thinking obedient part to come out, often not even knowing what it is doing. The perpetrators punish the parts who refuse to obey by hurting them badly, then putting them (that is, the child's body) in an actual garbage dump full of filth and feces. The perpetrators call these "garbage kids" (or "rubbish kids" in the UK).

This garbage dump is replicated internally. These parts, when found, can be very helpful in the healing process, as they have courage and fight hard not to obey the abusers.

Inner self-helpers

Many systems have parts who act as inner self-helpers, giving various kinds of care and nurturing to the other parts. Sometimes these parts are self-created; at other times they are parts who have abandoned their assigned jobs to take care of others inside. They can be very helpful in the healing process.

Floater parts

During severe abuse, many parts are frequently split off during a single event. There are parts who appear to the survivor to be able to float around the location of the child's body without residing in the body. The abuser groups are aware of the existence of these parts and call them "floaters." I have heard repeatedly of floaters seeing and hearing what is going on behind the scenes, things that can't be seen from the body's viewpoint. In some cases, they inform the part who is "out" in the body of what they see going on. In other cases, they keep quiet unless asked by the therapist or other parts of the system. I met one floater who claimed to travel great distances. Perhaps this is what the military organizations that studied "remote viewing" were working with.

I don't know the physics of this, but I have had enough experience of talking with floaters to know they are real. Survivors may have their own terms for them, such as "drifters." The abusers frequently try to gather in any floaters that may have been created during an abusive episode, as they know that floaters can interfere with the programming attempts. One survivor I knew would deliberately split off floaters who had the self-assigned role of holding onto the truth and imparting it to her later, or sometimes during an event in which the abusers were trying to deceive her.

Besides the floater parts who are simply observers of events, there can be many floaters who hold emotions. I have also heard of floaters who can act in the outside world even though invisible, for example breaking objects to distract abusers. Researchers have discovered that the supposedly ghostly entities called poltergeists, who do such things as move objects around and break dishes, usually manifest themselves around disturbed young people, primarily women. Perhaps they are floaters.

Floaters can be very helpful during the healing process, and I have found myself asking a client to inquire about floaters' knowledge when going through a traumatic memory, so that all aspects of the event can be included. To fully resolve infant memories, the floaters must be invited back into the body and to share their perceptions and emotions with the rest of the system. Floaters must be included for full integration.

Record keeper parts

Every victim of mind control programming has internal record keepers trained by perpetrators at a very early age. File keepers, librarians, and record keepers are some of the job titles given to these parts. They may have memorized entire conversations word for word in order to be able to repeat them back. I find that when a victim is working through a memory, they are able to repeat all words that were spoken, which is especially important since the program instructions are given in words.

The records these parts may have include:

- A copy of the victim's "black book" about his or her training experiences
- The memories of training experiences
- A record of all traumatic memories, including those abuse memories that were not part of formal training
- A record of all insiders, their locations, and their jobs.

Getting the record keepers to work with you can speed up therapy and make things intelligible.

Internal programmers or switch controllers

Switch controllers (also known as internal programmers) turn "programs" on and off by internal switches and buttons that have specific effects, like putting parts to sleep or making them suicidal or creating hallucinations. They are mid-age children who were placed in physical locations with these switches and control boards where they were trained to respond to cues and do their jobs. They may never have seen the actual outside world other than these places. They usually don't know what the switches they control do, although they may know the names of the programs they are turning on and off. They only know that they must do their jobs immediately when given the signal to do so. Signals to them may be external (from a perpetrator group member) or internal (such as some other part pushing a button connected to a wire). It is likely that those trained in later generations have some kind of computer program simulation rather than physical switches.

Gatekeepers

Gatekeepers hold in or release inside people. They act on instructions but have some latitude to make decisions if they are not being told directly what to do. Generally, a gatekeeper does not allow most trained parts "out" into the body unless given a special signal, such as a touch by someone else's hand on the left shoulder combined with the name of the part who is called for.

Pain holder parts

These are usually very young infants. Some hold physical pain. The pain for a victim never stops. Some victims are given diseases to weaken them and keep them in pain. Particular pain holder parts may hold pain in different body locations, or different kinds of pain (such as electroshock, dull ache, sharp stabbing, the sensation of being raped). This pain can be drawn upon by the punisher parts, who send it to the front people or others who have disobeyed the abusers.

Certain parts, such as soldiers and sexual masochists, are not supposed to feel actual pain, so pain holders (who may be sub-parts within them) hold the pain for them.

Some pain holders are specialized for holding emotional pain. Particular ones may hold despair, sadness, anger, frustration, anxiety, etc. These feelings are generally held in and not experienced by the front people, but they may be drawn upon to punish, just like the physical pain. The abusers may give anger to perpetrator parts or despair to the front people (to motivate a suicide attempt) when the group needs it. When a survivor puts together the memory of an episode of abuse, they may feel the pain consciously for the first time.

Some hold empathic pain for other people who are suffering or being hurt. When this pain is kept separate, perpetrator parts can do their jobs without feeling the pain of those they hurt. To help perpetrator parts stop doing these jobs, the healing system can share the empathic pain with them.

Programs and jobs for use in Satanic or Luciferian rituals

For a ritual, there may be a three-day preparation period. Parts are trained not to sleep or eat during this time. This weakening of the body makes them more susceptible to influences during the ritual. If your client is not eating or sleeping, you might look at a ritual calendar to see whether a ritual date is coming up.

For the ritual itself, parts to be victimized are trained to hold back urine and feces, to keep still and silent, not to run, and not to feel pain. In preparation for perpetration, parts are trained to use a knife for killing or dissection of a body (usually for consumption by the group in a ritual). Stella Katz (in *Healing the Unimaginable*) writes of a category of insider called "the Touch block." Besides killing and dissection, these trained parts may have the job of performing self-harm, usually as punishment for disobedience. The part receiving the pain feels it; the part doing the cutting or burning does not. This self-mutilation is different from non-programmed cutting where the person is trying to calm themselves and drive away emotional pain.

Some parts are trained to speak occult languages such as Enochian. I met one such child part who could only speak rapid Enochian, and who wrote in "mirror writing." I had to use a mirror to read what she was trying to tell me. Of course, a survivor who comes from another country may have parts who only know the language of the country where they lived in childhood. You may need to find an internal translator.

"Demon" parts

"Demons" and "devils" within a survivor are usually small child parts, split off at ages three to five, costumed and taught to make demon sounds by larger (adult) demon impersonators. They may have the names of demons found in ancient books. They have been taught no one will ever want them. They may have been taught they will harm anyone they speak with. If you try to banish them, they will go into hiding, or they may retaliate by destabilizing the client. Some Christian writers on this topic have said that you can tell real demons from trained parts by such things as recoiling from hearing the name of Jesus. In my experience, this only means that the ones who seem more real are better trained or are better actors.

"Animal" parts

Parts who believe themselves to be animals (or chimeras, half-animal and half-human) are used for doing what those animals do. Horses run fast, cats sneak out at night, dogs beg and come when called, snakes do dances at rituals. These parts are trained by being costumed, put in cages with animals, told they are that kind of animal, and only fed when they behave like that animal. One system's record keeper parts believed themselves to be orcas and were actually trained in a tank with orcas. They believed they couldn't speak.

Witches, psychics, and spiritual leaders

Because of experience and an interest since childhood, I have attempted to keep up with the developments in the field of parapsychology or extrasensory perception, and I believe these are genuine abilities possessed to some extent by all mammals including human beings. The organized perpetrator groups generally know about these abilities and utilize them in various ways. Sophisticated perpetrator groups, such as military agencies, assess children for known ESP abilities (telepathy, "remote viewing" capability, etc.). Those found to have such abilities are trained to use them on behalf of the group.

Ritually abusive groups create parts known as "witches" whose abilities are used to curse people, make predictions, assess victims for abilities, tell the group where to act (for evil or good) in the world. Parts with this training may believe they can kill with their minds, as this has been simulated in childhood. A child is told to kill someone by using their mind, then the target person falls to the ground and appears to be dead. However, parts called witches can disobey and curse the wrong person, and the group will not know.

Some parts of a survivor, whether or not they are trained, can use their psychic abilities to see inside other people and whom they can trust.

Ghosts and aliens and spirits

Do not panic if your client talks about a ghost or a spirit being within them. They may well have a part who believes itself to be a ghost or a spirit. Ghosts and other incorporeal entities are insider parts who were led to believe they do not belong to the body. When they are made (split off from other parts), the body is under the influence of anesthetic drugs, which make these apparently nonhuman parts unable to feel anything in the body. This helps them believe they do not belong to that body. Sometimes these parts represent suicide programs (internal homicide)— "kill this traitor's body." Sometimes they hold knowledge that they supposedly can't disclose because they can't speak. Sometimes they check up on and discipline the system leaders. You won't get to these for a long time; they are hidden and may be outside the primary system structure, designed to terrorize others in the system if those within the structure are disobedient. The most helpful approach is to prove to these parts that they are in the body. You can, for example, write something on the hand of another part, then invite the "spirit" to come out and look at their own hand, which will have that writing on it.

Reactivators of programs

Perpetrator groups need to have a way to reactivate any programs that have been deactivated through a survivor's healing process. They create reactivator parts for this purpose. Some of these insiders are instructed to take and hide a part of a training memory. In some cases, the reactivator gets to choose what part of the memory they will hide. In other cases, there is a word spoken or a symbol shown to the reactivator during the memory, to identify what memory it belongs to. These parts are hidden, and their job is to keep this piece of memory separate, so that if the survivor puts the training memory together, the piece is not included.

Whole groups of reactivator parts may be hidden. Their portion may be words, incidental details, emotion, or physical pain. These parts are brought out when the perpetrator group reaccesses the survivor to find out what happened to a program that isn't working correctly. They tell the perpetrators their part and the training is repeated. The reactivator parts also have the job of letting the perpetrators know that a particular memory has been worked on; by giving the perpetrator group their piece of memory, the group can know what training of theirs was disabled and can repeat the training to make the program work again. In some systems, other insiders are trained to put their piece on an internal turntable that will regrow the program. I don't know just how this works, but it reactivates the program. It may be related to the purpose of spinning. To destroy a program permanently, it is necessary to put together all training memories for this program and include every single part of those memories, especially the pieces held by the reactivators.

Paired programs

Programs are often taught in pairs of opposites, in which only one pole is activated at a time. Some examples are sleep/insomnia, eat/don't eat, tell (report the truth to abusers)/don't tell (outsiders), run/don't run, and die/don't die. If you, the therapist, are ready to work with the client on undoing one of these programs, you should search for its opposite as well. It is probably found within the same training session or series of trainings.

Recognizing programming

You can recognize specific programs by their effects. It is important to know that the part "out" in the world is not the one in control of programmed behavior. If, for example, your client has been cutting their arms, it may not do any good to ask the part who cuts about why they do it, because they don't know. However, this part or the front part may be able to ask inside to get information from other parts.

Program triggers

When a program is installed, it comes with triggers that perpetrator group members can use to activate it. A family member, for example, can send a victim a birthday card with beautiful white roses on it—and shortly after receiving this card, the victim makes a suicide attempt. Triggers can be visual, auditory, or kinesthetic (through touch). Perpetrator group members are placed in leadership positions in churches or similar groups in order to send messages through hand signals or facial signals or words. Zoom gives them a helpful platform. I realized that one client was a survivor by seeing her respond to a touch trigger for "forget", which her hand did on her own face. If you know hand signals, foot signals, or facial signals, you might observe parts trying to send messages to you via these. Many sight triggers just look like normal movements: brushing hair off the face, blinking a certain number of times, touching a left shoulder, holding the hands in a particular position. Certain words that are normally innocuous may trigger programs.

Turning programs on and off (and down)

Programs are activated in a survivor by remembering the abuse, talking about the abuse, everyday accidental triggers (words, touches, sounds, sights), deliberate triggers sent or given by perpetrator group members, events, and dates. Sometimes the same trigger will activate or turn off different programs in different survivors, although I have found some consistency among clients abused by the same or related perpetrator groups. Many programs have "off" triggers as well as "on" triggers. If you know the triggers, you can turn a program off, but this should only be used in an emergency because it might make your client suspect you are a perpetrator. Programs turned off can always be turned on again, so turning them off (especially without the permission of all parts of your client) is only a temporary measure. You can only permanently deactivate a program by putting together the memories that created the program, with all involved parts. (See Chapter 8 of this book for more detail.) You can ask the parts of the person in charge of a program to turn it off, or if they are afraid to do that, to temporarily turn it down so its effects are barely noticeable (but it will need to be addressed more thoroughly later). Programs involving self-harm or pain are good targets for this.

Attaching programs to places or events

Perpetrator groups can attach programs to events or places. For example, a program may be activated by entering the therapist's office. Programs can be attached to one another. For example, if a therapist attempts to undo the "suicide" program it activates the "paranoia" program. If the therapist attempts to undo the "paranoia" program, it activates the "run away" program. "What will happen if …?" is a very useful question. If current contact with perpetrators is suspected, you might discuss such linkages by telephone with internal programmers before an appointment. Some parts of the client may be able to make a "wiring diagram" of how the programs are attached to one another, and then you can together dismantle the programs in the order that will do the least harm. It is current abusers who create the linkages. (See p. 161 of *Healing the Unimaginable* and Chapter 8 of this book.)

CHAPTER 5

Stabilization and internal safety

S urvivors of organized mind-controlling abuse, like any abuse survivors, sometimes experience unintended posttraumatic triggering: Something reminds the survivor of a trauma, and the survivor experiences a partial flashback, emotional state, or body memory (body symptoms that come from a memory.) People who have had traumatic experiences are often destabilized by traumatic intrusions, such as flashbacks, nightmares, body memories, and emotional states of sadness, anxiety, and despair. Self-harm is a method some trauma survivors use to try to reduce these intrusions. Suicide attempts can also be a way to flee these unbearable states. However, when a therapist's usual stabilization methods are ineffective, it may be because the client has a structured personality system acting on programming. Survivors' flooding of feelings, flashbacks, physical pain, suicide attempts, or self-harm are often deliberately created by inside parts doing their assigned jobs, usually of punishing the survivor for disobedience.

Programmed triggering

A mind control survivor client may experience programmed triggering from various sources. It may be set off by an external cue like a hand or facial signal from an abuser group member or a letter or phone call from home. The cue usually gives a reminder about loyalty, or not remembering, or that the group knows everything the survivor does, and it might tell inner parts to punish the survivor for disobedience. Programmed triggering may also be set off by the date, as some parts have been trained to do a job on a particular date. The job may be to attend an event or meeting, or prepare for that event, or go somewhere to receive instructions. It might be to create a physical illness to debilitate the survivor. Then there is programmed punishment triggering: The survivor disobeys the rules of an abuser or an organized abusive group, and inner parts punish with reminders of a trauma.

Programmed internal punishments

Organized criminal groups set up security programming in victims' personality systems so that if a survivor or a therapist makes discoveries about the personality system or memories, the survivor is likely to destabilize. A huge portion of programming is about the group's security. Most punishment consists of releasing parts of traumatic memories (such as overwhelming emotions, physical pain, scary sights, and scary sounds) to the front person. These are usually warnings of what might happen if the person continues to disobey the abusers.

All these abuser groups have the same basic rules: Be obedient and loyal to past and present abusers, maintain a façade of normalcy (or of craziness if you've been discarded for saying too much), don't get close to any outsiders, and don't disclose anything about the abuse. Breaking these rules brings on punishment by parts who have the job of punishing disobedience. It is wise to slow down disclosures if punishment is frequent or severe. It is important to develop a bond of trust with the leaders of the personality system, the ones who may have the authority to stop or reduce the punishment.

The following is a partial list of programmed internal punishments that make the victim unable to function normally:

- Various kinds of pain, which are actually punisher-controlled bodily flashbacks from memories
- Pseudo-seizures or head jerks, resulting from electroshock memories being administered as punishment
- Bodily symptoms that resemble illnesses
- Seeing horrendous scenes, which are controlled visual flashbacks of horrible memories
- Hallucinations, usually of the presence of perpetrators
- Nightmares
- Paranoid delusions, such as believing that a bomb will go off in the body
- Intermittent learning disabilities, or scrambling of sensory information, distorting what people say
- Extreme depression, mood swings, and flooding of unpleasant emotions.

How most internal punishments and warnings work

The inside part with the job of punishing accesses a piece of a traumatic memory, such as the feeling of despair or the sight of someone dressed up as Satan or God, or the sound of a baby crying, or the sensation of pain. This is probably done by finding the inner person who holds this sensation. Wendy Hoffman in *From the Trenches* (Hoffman & Miller, 2018, p. 124) says that the part in charge of the punishment "is like a conductor of an orchestra. He calls out the musicians who play instruments but does not play an instrument him or herself." Spinner parts spin the piece of memory out to the rest of the system so that the front person and others will experience it as if is happening to them in the present. Even the bizarre symptoms come from memories of bizarre events and are deliberately designed.

Pain management

A survivor wrote to me about how pain worked in her system (note that pain here is a generic term for all kinds of discomfort, emotional as well as physical):

> There are several groups regarding pain: (1) "Pain-Holders" (2) "Pain-Givers" and (3) "Pain-Receivers" and (4) "Pain-Managing Parts."

Only the Pain-Receivers experience pain unmitigated as the Pain-Holders and Pain-Givers are involved with the pain dispensation, so don't feel it, and the Pain-Managers have learnt how to manage pain, especially if mixed with sexual arousal, or take the pain for some religious "integrity" issue where those would not ever want to crack for the sake of loyalty to the true God.

So, the Pain-Holders have all the knowledge and equipment to do the deed, but they don't do it themselves—they merely direct matters and aren't the recipients. They were often forced to be Leaders inside too. There is a Back-Up called "Full Stop!" as the abusers ordered her to "stop things going worse if the insider leaders were ever foolish enough to risk defying us. They sure know what would happen to them if they did. All the pain they make sure happens would come onto their shoulders and each would be killed slowly, with their eyeballs and entrails pulled out and crushed, and those Leaders would be replaced, then raped from morning through to the next morning, each day until they expire. No one stays clean if given enough incentive ..."

The Pain-Givers go to these Pain-Holder parts and present the case as to why the pain needs to be inflicted, if it seems a bit different/beyond their usual role, and then they can do it if given approval.

The Pain-Receivers who are the targets for the pain have been forced into roles. Some are masochistic in outlook, where they are taught to feel helpless and unable to do anything about any undesirable situation. They experience the fullness of the pain. These struggle with wanting to die and can feel pretty depressed with every moment being like agony when in considerable pain. The Pain-Receivers were told by the abusers repeatedly "You have to suffer the full brunt as you defied us and you must see that there is really no point in attracting that sort of punishment by any of you trying to get free. You see how painful and useless that notion is! You must make sure we get told who inside was being rebellious, then you all have to take the result!"

When you as the therapist realize that all your client's destabilizing symptoms are caused by parts deliberately sabotaging the person's health, it is tempting to try to help the parts in the personality system who are experiencing the symptoms battle with the punishers, whom they see as the "bad guys." Don't do this! It fosters internal splitting instead of resolving internal conflicts. Instead, you need to reassure, reason with, and educate the parts who do their jobs, and, even more important, the parts with authority over the rest of the system.

Internal disasters

Your client may experience some kind of internal disaster, in which the structures in the internal world are destroyed. Abusers simulate each disaster (a tidal wave, a flood, a fire, an earthquake) in childhood with a model of the inner world. At the same time, the child is put through a similar experience. I have known several survivors who have gone through a house fire. A flood is simulated with a fire hose, an earthquake by putting the child on a structure that shakes and collapses. Internal disasters put the whole personality system into disarray and it needs to be rebuilt. The plan (and training) of the perpetrators is that the victim will return to them to have them put it in order again when such a disaster has happened.

Programmed behaviors that punish the victim

Some parts are trained to punish the body in specific ways (cutting, burning, or scratching), sometimes carving symbols into the flesh. The part who carries out the action may or may not be the one who initiates it. The part who does it may not feel the harm; the pain is carried by other insider parts. The part who does it is generally not responsible for it but is made to act that way by other parts with more authority. Some systems have parts trained to injure the body as a punishment or in response to a cue. Or to cause a car accident. In survivors of ritual abuse and mind control, self-harm and suicide attempts are often not a result of despair but programmed behaviors, internal punishments for disobedience, administered by enforcer parts. These are trained child parts who fear death or torture to themselves or others if they don't do their jobs.

Many survivors have programs for eating disorders: overeating, starving, and bulimia. Anorexia, like a suicide attempt, can get a victim into hospital, where it is easier for abusers to get hold of them. Other parts have the job of attempting suicide, which may well get them into hospital even if it is not serious.

One seriously dangerous program is for internal homicide, that is, one part trying to kill the body that houses the rest of the system. This can be quite dangerous, as some parts may be ordered to kill the body, often believing they are not part of the body. This can be triggered by the perpetrator group if the person is a serious threat to its security.

Self-harm training

In survivors of ritual abuse and mind control, self-harm is not just a spontaneous self-calming behavior. Rather, certain inside parts are trained to harm the body in specific ways if the person is disloyal or discloses secrets. For example, a child is branded with a pentagram, told it marks her as a servant of Satan, and if she is disloyal, she must make this mark on her own body to prove her loyalty. Introject parts of the perpetrators must do what those actual perpetrators did. Patterns of cuts and burns give visible messages that the person has been abused by a cult group, so that local cult members, such as patients and staff members in a psychiatric hospital, can get hold of the victim and take them for retraining. Some victims are trained to experience sexual pleasure with self-harm, and it can become an addiction. I have also known a survivor who had parts specifically trained to split off copies of themselves through engaging in self-harm, thus creating countless backups. Perpetrator group members, including other programmed survivors, can (knowingly or unknowingly) give cues to trigger self-harming behavior.

Suicide, and suicide attempt training

According to the Extreme Abuse Survey (http://eassurvey.wordpress.com/extreme-abuse-survey-final-results/), ritual abuse and mind control survivors attempted suicide more often than extreme abuse survivors who did not report ritual abuse or mind control, but their success rate was no higher. Suicide attempts, like self-harm, are punishments. Perpetrator groups put a lot of time and effort into training their victims, and do not like them to die or to draw attention through a successful suicide. Survivors usually have a "don't die" program, usually involving fear of going to hell. See Wendy Hoffman's essay "To Die or Not To Die" in *From the Trenches* (Hoffman & Miller, 2018, pp. 170–172). The perpetrators train children to attempt suicide in very specific ways (for example, to take a few pills less than a lethal amount). As with self-harm, perpetrators or other survivors can give cues to trigger this behavior.

We need to develop the ability to assess the degree of risk for our survivor clients. We must not push them too early into decisions that will imperil them to the extent that they die at their own hands or the hands of the perpetrator group. We must become accustomed to some degree of risk, which is inevitable with survivor clients, both because of their suicide programming and the possibility that they will be murdered (often disguised as suicide) if they disclose too many perpetrator secrets.

Risks of hospitalization

Therapists often overreact to self-harm events by trying to get their clients into psychiatric hospitals where safety is someone else's responsibility. This is also a goal of many abuser groups, as they want disobedient members in hospitals where they can access them. Much effort is put by perpetrators into infiltrating psychiatric hospitals. Perhaps a few psychiatric hospitals are safe, but the one in my city certainly wasn't. There was a cult van that openly picked up survivors at the front door (where patients went out to smoke) at dinner time. There were rituals and cult-led fake therapy groups in the basement at night.

Cult members can also deliberately injure a survivor, making it look like self-harm, in the hope that the survivor's therapist will see the harm and hospitalize the client. A client once came into my office bleeding from her arm, but she immediately told me that the cult members had ambushed her on her way to our appointment, and she hadn't done it herself. I believed her. Please do not hospitalize a victim for trivial reasons such as minor self injury or suicidal ideation. If there is serious injury that must be treated in a hospital, a general hospital may be less risky for survivors than a psychiatric one. There is a reason why so many suicides happen right after hospitalization.

Booby traps—mild and serious

"Booby traps" within a survivor are set off if the person tries to break the code of conduct. Some are designed to kill; some are designed to make the person seem insane and tell wild stories; some make the system crash and the person lose all memory. One very bad booby trap is an overwhelming feeling of guilt and depression, feelings so overwhelming that the person gets trapped in the emotion. These emotions come from events in childhood: the death of a loved person or pet, or abandonment and being told they are unlovable even by God. Perpetrators lie to the victims and tell them that the "angel of suicide," previously discussed in Chapter 3 of this book, also known as the angel of the sunset, can stop this pain.

Internal homicide training

Another serious risk is internal homicide. As I wrote previously, the perpetrator groups do not easily give up on a victim after expending years of training on them. But they believe they own their victims, and indeed everyone in their bloodline. Their security comes ahead of the life of those victims. Certain parts of each victim are trained to believe they do not belong to the body and will not die when the body dies.

Parts who harm or try to kill the body often don't feel pain, and believe they aren't part of the body. Because of that mind control, they believe they can jump off buildings or set fire to their bodies without the supposedly body-free parts being harmed. But this programming isn't triggered by the group until the perpetrator group has given up on using the person and considers the person a serious security threat.

With someone with DID or OSDD, it is not easy to tell whether there is a serious suicide risk. One part can have a pleasant therapy session, then another part can try to jump off the building, or think about doing so. You need to assess whether the group might want the person to die, risking a police investigation. If you come to know there are parts who seriously want to kill the body, which they believe isn't theirs, you can show these parts that they are in the same body with the others. For example, draw on the body's hand, then ask the parts who are supposed to harm or kill the body to come out, move that hand, and look at it as they move it.

Pacing the therapy

Don't hurry and don't investigate; slow down to stabilize. You are a therapist, not a detective. The client may assume your purpose is to find out secrets. Reassure them that it isn't, that your purpose is trying to help them take charge of their own life. Don't let detective parts of your survivor client hurry you into opening up their memories too fast, as this is likely to provoke both internal and external punishment. Do not rush to find things out before the inside parts in charge have developed sufficient trust. If you push for disclosures or memories, this will provoke parts to do their jobs of destabilization and reporting to abusers. Delay memory work until internal leaders are ready to permit it. Your aim must be to develop rapport with those internal leaders. But you'll get nowhere if you delay until there is complete stability.

CHAPTER 6

Working with the personality system

Internal hierarchies and leaders

Most (but not all) organized personality systems have internal hierarchies, which may mirror the structure of the abuser groups. When there is a hierarchy, you can work with the internal leaders who can shut down any programming until you are able to work with the actual memories that created the programs. When there is little or no hierarchy, lots of internal children may continue to do their jobs, believing in the lies the abusers told them and fearing abusers who are long gone. The survivor needs to form a new internal coalition that can seek out these child parts and reeducate them internally and/or work through their training memories. But, as hierarchies are the most common, I shall focus on them.

Bosses (higher-ups)

The higher-ups in a hierarchical system may have impressive names and titles. One Nazi-created system, for example, had a series of Hitlers, with the one at the top being the "real Hitler." A Satanic system had a series of Satans, with various adjectives attached, the first few layers numbered Satan 1 through 9, and then the Most High Satan. Thirteen layers are more common. Many bosses may have the names of actual perpetrators (trainers or programmers) who were in the abused child's life.

Enforcers, soldiers, and guards

In the internal world, enforcers administer punishments when the person has broken the perpetrators' rules. They are obeying the orders of their bosses, the higher-ups. If the person is considering breaking the rules (such as telling a therapist something important), there are parts who issue internal threats regarding what will happen (externally as well as internally) if the rules are violated. In some systems, there has been systematic training of child soldiers who then become soldier parts. While they have internal jobs, they might be called on at some time to become actual fighters in the external world. Some are trained to use weapons, including guns. They are highly trained in loyalty, much like real adult soldiers. They may believe they have killed other soldiers, as this has been simulated during their training. Remember that most of the internal parts have not aged with the body. Internal bosses are usually aged twelve or thirteen, while programmed soldiers and enforcers may be younger than that.

Internal leaders are crucial to recovery

The internal bosses and their enforcers issue threats when the survivor disobeys the rules, and administer punishment for disobedience or disclosures, commanding flashbacks or self-harm or ordering programs to be turned on. To really change things, those parts in charge, at the top of the hierarchy, must decide to make a break for freedom. Those parts, who rarely (if ever) come out in everyday life, need to learn about how the survivor's life circumstances have changed so that in adulthood freedom is possible. The internal leaders also need to discover that they were deceived by the mind controllers, that their power is only internal, and that they do not deserve lifelong slavery as puppets of the perpetrator group. Even if a system has no hierarchy, there are parts in charge, and they must make the decision to work for healing.

When I met "Sally," she had been very dysfunctional for years and was on a disability pension, living in noisy, lice-infested, low-cost housing for the mentally ill. She tells her own story in Chapter 6 of *Becoming Yourself* (Miller, 2014). Her higher-ups prided themselves in tormenting her kind therapist of seven years by sending her dozens of emails each week and making Sally repeatedly relive painful body memories and/or harm herself during therapy sessions. I saw Sally as a temporary vacation fill-in for her regular therapist, and when she began to do this in our session, I recognized this behavior as programmed and ordered whoever inside Sally was making this happen to stop it immediately. Shocked, she did as she was told. Not long afterward, when Sally made a serious suicide attempt, her therapist finally gave up and told Sally she must choose another therapist. Sally asked the therapist to refer her to me. Her higher-up parts understood firmness. Sally and I worked together for many years. By the end, when I retired, Sally was working full time, living in co-op housing, and doing very well. She contributed to both my books, *Healing the Unimaginable* (2012a, pp. 58–66) as "Old Lady" (which is what her child parts called her) and Chapter 6, pp. 71–81 of *Becoming Yourself.*

At one point, I had an email conversation with her higher-up parts about how her system worked. They told me that

> We were created to keep everyone [inside] in line so that they would remain loyal to the organizations who made us. They were our family, not the parents, and we owed our lives to them; they were our leaders, fathers, mothers, military trainers, confidantes and family. They would always protect us if we obeyed them and were loyal. From the body's first anointment at birth, we had to keep the body in line via the little ones being told to follow commands, acting like robots for us, and thus not asking or whining or thinking, just doing regardless of the consequences.

Sally's primary abuser group was an extreme right-wing one, apparently involving (in Canada) the Ku Klux Klan and the Nazis. Sally was born into one of their families. Her higher-ups had done an excellent job of keeping her in line.

Trainers' words to higher-ups

Sally's higher-ups wrote to me what their trainers had said to them in childhood: "You belong to us, you are ours, you are property, to be owned only by us and for our use and no other." "We will tell you what to do and when." There was a big emphasis on instant unthinking obedience. "Obey or be killed. Obey or suffer. Obey and do." "Do not think—just do it." This was combined with encouragement for her as a white child to become both loyal to the abusers and very tough and strong. "Obey us and be strong and do not let any outsider fool you into believing their lies. You are free with us not with them, you don't need to think, for we think for you and for your safety and your power, so that you may have power over life itself, and the blood of all humanity, and animals." "Obeying and being able to take pain via training makes you stronger and more determined to follow our light, the light of darkness, the way of truth, of light, of power, and the superiority and power of the Aryan race over all humans and life. You are superior and will honor us till death or be called a traitor and die with the outsiders in mind, spirit, and body. We will make it so."

There were threats, and promises of rewards for obedience, the rewards being only the lack of severe negative consequences. "For your work, little ones, you will be rewarded by not being harmed, thrown into prison, into caves or coffins or killed or tortured or have your friends killed or sacrificed." "You will listen or be punished and sent to hell, for God is not the leader here, we are—the Luciferians, SS, and KKK." "Do not deceive us or we will find you and bring you back or dispose of you or make you self-destruct."

Facts about higher-ups

It is important for therapists to realize that just because an insider is named Hitler or Satan or the name of someone who abused the child does not mean that part wants to be like that person. To really help your client change things, you (the therapist) need to work your way up to the top of the hierarchy and talk with those in charge. The higher-up parts, who rarely, if ever, come out in everyday life, may not know about how the survivor's life circumstances have changed. Many higher-ups have no experience in the real world. They are typically aged twelve or thirteen. They do not know that the body is an adult now, or that they are (in some cases) far away from the abusers. Higher-ups often do not realize that their power is only internal, over inside parts in the same body with them. Quite often they hate the abusers and are waiting for a chance to escape them and even get back at them. As you talk with other parts of the personality system, the higher-ups watch how you treat their subordinates. If you are kind, if you listen, if you are unlike the abusers, the higher-ups take note of it.

Stopping programmed symptoms (warnings or punishments)

When you see punishment being administered or hear that threats are being made internally, you need to negotiate with the insiders *causing* the flashback or self-harm or hallucinations, not the ones *experiencing* it. Recognize that these parts are not really malevolent; they are just doing what they have to in order to avoid what they have been told will happen if they don't do their jobs. Ask to speak to the one who ordered the pain, showed the horrible picture, made the person dizzy, made them sleepy, or made them want to cut. Then reassure that internal person that they are not in trouble and ask what message they are giving to the client's front person, and what rule might have been broken.

Every symptom is a warning to the parts not to be disloyal to the perpetrators. Look for the perpetrators' threat behind the warning. Ask the one who ordered or administered the symptom, "What are you afraid might happen if she breaks that rule?" Bring the threat out into the open. Suggest that actual words in the head would be more effective to convey the message that the pain or other symptom was trying to give. Promise to listen to spoken warnings and pass them on to the parts who have broken the group's rules. Remember that everyone in your client's body has a boss who is listening and considering what you say.

What are you to do when your client winces or groans (indicating they are being punished with pain) or self-harms in your office during an appointment? Giving memory pain to other parts is also self-harm, in a way, so whether or not the body is actually being harmed afresh, you can say, "Hey! You're not allowed to hurt bodies in here. I don't do it and you aren't allowed to either. Stop it!" Then follow this with saying more softly—"You aren't in trouble. You just need to learn the rules of my office." Even internal punishers expect punishment! The words "in trouble" are words used frequently by perpetrators, so hearing they are not in trouble is important to victims. Now reiterate the rules of your office, including "Don't harm bodies."

If a symptom's purpose is to warn the client about you, you can speak to whichever part gave the warning, and ask, "What do you think I'm trying to do?" Now enter a dialogue with that part. For example, in response to certain reactions of the client, you might say something like "Do you think I know too much about these matters? … But you need a therapist who knows what kind of thing you're dealing with. You've already tried therapists who didn't understand these abuses." Or "I learned about this from my clients/ from a book/ from a workshop. Not from you. I already knew it before you said anything, so you shouldn't be in trouble for telling me." Or "I am not part of the abuser group. Your protectors can watch me and see whether I behave like those people." Sometimes parts of a client hear you mention something about ritual abuse or mind control and think one of their parts must have disclosed this information, so they punish the body. You can say, "Don't punish *them* for what *I* said. I didn't learn it from you."

Making your way up a hierarchy

If a part considers stopping their job or being disloyal to the abusers, they may hear a voice threatening them. When you see your client pause and appear to be listening to something other than you, they may be hearing an internal warning or a threat. Ask what the client is listening to. If it's a voice, ask what it's saying. Then ask to talk to the voice. Remember that even if it appears to be an internal copy of an abuser, or a fearsome demon, it is a part just like everyone else inside, and it therefore has a connection to the person's true self. Ask its age. Make your conversation appropriate for that age. Do not ask its name. Abusers use the names of parts to call them out for punishment.

If you convince this voice you are safe, another voice may appear with a different threat or causing a different symptom. Ask to talk to the new one, then do this repeatedly until you get to someone with some authority. Get to know each one until it is replaced by its boss or backup. The process takes time. Be content not to know many things for a long time.

Reach out with compassion towards increasingly higher levels of parts within the person. Ask to speak with those parts who make threats or give punishments such as pain. Be curious but gentle even when firm; don't interrogate or confront. Demonstrate your understanding that parts may have jobs that they have been forced to do. Listen to the client's pacing. Get to know each part until it is replaced (in the front) by its boss or backup. Tell them you know that their trust must be earned and that you do not expect them to trust you, but they should keep observing you and draw their own conclusions. Work to get them to think for themselves.

Ask about what they've been told about people like you. Clarify your role. "You think I'm here to get you to tell all your memories? No, that's not my purpose at all. My purpose is to help all of you to have a better life, a life you may want, and to be in charge of your own life rather than the slave of someone else." And if a part appears to be afraid of you, "What do you expect me to do? … You think I'll abuse you? Why do you think that? … Did someone tell you I'd do that? … Did someone else do those things to you? … Ask the parts who know me whether I've ever done that."

Dialogue that exposes the deceptions

As you talk with parts who have jobs, don't argue with them, but join them, agree, and point out where and how they are absolutely correct. You can also ask (repeatedly) "Is that right? Huh. Who told you that?" or "Hmm. I wonder when was the first time you heard that statement?" or "Mmm. That's interesting. I wonder who on the outside of you says such things?" or even "You know, you weren't born with that belief, so how did you get that belief?" Stay objective, neutral, and matter of fact—and curious, interested, and wanting to understand. You can see some long examples of this in pages 95–104 of my book *Becoming Yourself* or my essay "Dialogue with the higher-ups" in Ralf Vogt's book *Perpetrator Introjects* (2012b, pp. 111–132.)

Topics for dialogue

The topics for dialogue with the parts who have jobs include what they believe or were taught about outsiders like you, why they believe the group owns them, why they believe they have to obey such people, the truth of what they were taught, and possibilities for safety, protection, and freedom.

Watch your use of such trigger words as "safe," "free," truth," love," "escape," and other words you might want to use, however, as abusers may have reversed their meanings so that they mean their opposites to the survivor. You may need to find synonyms that have not been used by abusers.

I consulted with a client on behalf of that client's therapist, with the consultation question being "Is there programming?" The problem was that the client was not allowed to use the word "programming" and would have a strong negative response to that word. So I suggested to the client that we give this problem a new name, such as "Johnny." We had a conversation in which I would refer to "Johnny." The humor in this helped the client relax. We could talk about the subject matter without breaking the abuser group's rules about words.

Unmasking the deceptions

These parts are all children who have been deceived and tortured and threatened with extreme pain and death. So be gentle as you help them unmask their deceptions. Many parts may think they still live with abusers in their childhood home, because they have not come "out" into the world since childhood. Frequently update the whole system about time and place. There are various ways to help them realize that they have been deceived. An important one is to ask parts who know the truth about something to communicate it internally to those who don't. This encourages internal communication and is more effective than asking them to believe you.

If you discover a trick of the abusers, you can demonstrate a similar trick to one the abusers used, without abuse. For example, abusers use a mirror with a picture of a demon pasted onto it to convince a child that she or he is a demon. You can put a smiley face on a mirror and then take it off, so that the mirror shows the real face. If you are speaking to a part who believes it's in a different body, you can ask it to watch while you write on the hand of another part, then ask it to come out and view its own hand. You can have parts together view an event in which they had different parts (for example, the one a rat was put inside, and the one who believes she gave birth to the rat).

Effects of the dialogue

Sally's higher-ups gave me a list of effects of our dialogue. The first item was alerting the security system to turn on programs that could make Sally appear inaccessible, hostile, or overwhelmed. They told me not to be fooled by this. Because, according to Sally's higher-ups, that dialogue made the insiders, including the higher-ups, begin to think for them-selves and wonder about the answers to my questions and whether my statements were true. It shook the foundation of the beliefs indoctrinated into them. (Perhaps any statement of truth opens this door, no matter how much hostility it appears to provoke). That dialogue exposed the ways in which Sally's higher-ups had been deceived. It gave these insiders the opportunity to talk on an equal basis with someone kind and curious, as opposed to their abusers who gave orders and were cruel. It reduced Sally's dissociation by encouraging her insiders to obtain information from one another and from the front person. It made the apparently unemotional higher-ups aware of the emotional and physical pain that created them, which was still being held in the discarded and lower-down insiders. It made the loyal higher-ups begin to feel, or at least be aware of, the unmet needs, sadness, loss, and constant fear and anxiety expe-rienced by other insiders. It made memories of hurt insiders accessible to perpetrator insiders, which ended their desire to perpetrate. It helped parts stuck in the past become aware of present-day reality and gave hope for freedom and recovery in the present and future. It got the head of the system to engage and begin to think for himself. It gradually dissolved this part of Sally's programming. It connected parts of the person to their own spiritual essence and helped her regain control over her own life. All these wonderful things happened because of this dialogue!

Of course, this is not all the work you will do, as programming is very complex, but it is a good start. When you have worked with one hierarchy and its leaders, there may be more sections and parts to discover. But once you catch on to how programming works, you can help your client make faster progress in their healing.

Building inner community

It is important to remember that all parts, no matter what they have been told, are human: the infants from the foundation, the children who were given jobs, the adults who may have had to act in the world on behalf of the perpetrators, the adult front parts who have to cope with everyday life challenges. Each insider part began its "life" at the time of a major trauma and is stuck at the age of another major trauma during which it was replaced. We therapists must relate to them with this in mind. Each part is in some way connected to the core, a human soul, longing for connection and healing. No one inside is a "bad guy," no matter what they may have done. Those parts who enforce perpetrators' rules are working for the safety of the person or of other people. Some actual perpetrator adults do it to save their own children and other family members, choosing their family's safety over that of other victims, whom they may be ordered to harm. Of course, perpetrator groups are very deceptive, and the other people any victim may believe they are protecting may actually continue to be harmed. Abusers are liars.

Most engineered personality systems have internal leaders assigned by the perpetrators. Healing proceeds as these important parts decide to transform themselves and work on behalf of the person and against the goals of the perpetrator group. They can give orders to those under their authority, and they can learn to use their authority wisely and kindly. This can come naturally. Very often such parts know what kind of authorities they would have preferred to learn from, in contrast to their parents and programmers. Your client can gradually move towards an internal democracy in which the leaders in the governing council represent all parts' needs. They can research each group of insiders— their ages, likes and dislikes, needs. How could the system provide for their needs in the external world? In the inner world? Although an excellent outcome is to become one person rather than many scattered parts, there are plenty of steps along the way, and it is up to each survivor to discover what they are capable of achieving. Some survivors who achieve cooperative personality systems may prefer not to pursue integration, although integration sometimes gains its own momentum and proceeds anyway. Choosing not to integrate can work well if there is no perpetrator group continuing to interfere in the person's life, but it can be a handicap if perpetrators can call out parts.

Insiders often have names that reflect their roles in the abuse; they can choose different names. Costumed insiders can take off the costumes. Some parts may have been told by adult perpetrators to be copies of them (the abusive adults), and they need help to become kids again. You can ask parts to stop doing harmful jobs. You can ask parts to do their original jobs when they are helpful, such as putting away troubling memories or helping parts stuck in trauma to go to sleep temporarily until the system has time to help them more fully. Switch controllers and internal programmers can turn off programs and can provide a list of programs to be dismantled by working through the training memories. (See Chapter 8 for more about this.)

Giving insiders new jobs

As parts with jobs identify themselves and join the internal coalition for healing, they can choose new jobs. Trained parts are accustomed to having a purpose, even if that purpose is to further the aims of the perpetrator group. They still need a purpose, and a new job can provide it. The system can use insiders' job skills to assist in recovery. New jobs may resemble old jobs in terms of the skills required, but of course are for the purpose of helping the recovery process. For example:

- File keepers and librarians can keep traumatic and programming memories contained and organized (which they do anyway) and then bring them up when ready to process them
- Observers and recorders can watch the survivor's present life to make sure they are safe
- Spinners can spin away bad feelings and spin peaceful and calm feelings out into the system
- Pain holders can help reduce the pain of medical and dental appointments
- Soldier parts can get the body to exercise and to endure pain
- "Forget" program holders can make reporter parts forget anything they may have been trained to report.

It is important, however, to see what each part or group of parts is really like. For example, you might think "soldier" parts would be useful for doing difficult tasks. But soldiers are trained in instant obedience to perpetrators, so having them out in the world is risky. Garbage kids, however, are the ones who refused to act on their training, refused to do what the perpetrators told them to do, even at great personal cost. They are the ones your client wants for tasks that involve standing up to perpetrators. This is true even if their standing-up-to is silent, such as not telling how the person is disobeying the perpetrators.

Ways parts can improve their inner world

The imagination of your client's personality system will supply ways to improve the inner world that was initially installed by the perpetrators. Survivor Jen Callow's 2014 article "How I created my inner community" is an excellent example. You can see it in *Becoming Yourself* (Miller, 2014, pp. 151–154) or in *Healing the Unimaginable* (Miller, 2012a, pp. 272–275).

Some improvements I have heard from survivors include:

- Cutting wires and destroying control towers.
- Rescuing parts who are stuck in inner copies of the places where the abuse occurred: boxes, coffins, cages, cold basement rooms, garbage pits, bedrooms where a rapist found them.
- Giving inner kids their own rooms with locks on the inside and comfortable beds or couches.
- Making nurseries for babies, assigning internal caregivers, giving the infants stuffed animals, toys, blankets, pets.
- Creating new housing such as condominiums or tree houses or hidden places, whatever is most helpful.
- Making places for exercise, sports, and anger release.
- Allowing child parts to express themselves internally in art and play. Such expressive therapies are very helpful for traumatized children and will help parts who cannot speak about their traumatic experiences to release the emotions created by those experiences.
- Creating inner TV screens for safely viewing the outer world.

- Creating an inner movie of present-day life to update newly discovered insiders.
- Importing movie or TV or book characters as helpers, such as nannies, doctors, and nurses, or as surrogate new families replacing families of origin.

Ask, negotiate, command …

With some personality systems, asking and negotiating do not work, and verbal commands are necessary with some parts. This is because you are speaking with very young parts who are trained to respond only to commands, often phrased in a particular way. These parts are concrete and literalistic. They are not offended by commands. I think negotiation is preferable most of the time, but some of the time a command may be necessary. I have had clients ask me to phrase a request as a command in order that their literalistic parts will do what I ask.

"Turn it off"

The useful command "Turn it off!" can, with some systems, work to get programs temporarily turned off. Sometimes you need to add "in the name of Satan, whom I don't believe in." For example, "I command you in the name of Satan, whom I don't believe in, to stop, turn off, and put away the suicide program." If internal programmers are afraid to turn a program off, they can turn it down, so it is barely noticeable. And spinners can spin in the opposite direction, spinning the effects of the program back to the part it originally affected and away from the rest of the system. Of course, these are temporary measures, prior to the survivor coming to complete understanding of how and why the program was inserted.

Program codes

Program codes are sequences of letters and numbers that, when spoken or written correctly, will turn programs on or off or even destroy them. You may be able to obtain codes from the client's internal programmers. Internal programmers are kids who turn apparently electrical switches on and off in response to cues. Knowing codes and saying the "off" codes can help in undoing programming. It can neutralize programs so they do not get in the way of the therapy. This shortcut does not remove the trauma; it just temporarily keeps parts from doing their jobs. You can ask for program lists or charts with their codes (when you get that far and are planning systematic memory work). Much "deprogramming" by so-called experts is simply using such codes. It does not resolve the trauma. There is a long example of program codes on page 160 of *Healing the Unimaginable* (Miller, 2012a).

Using program triggers

The perpetrators design some programs so that only an external person can give the signal to turn them on and off. If you use triggers, especially without permission, parts may believe you are a perpetrator. But you and your client together can agree that you may do this in specific situations. Your client may have to tell you just what to say or do. For example, "No pain" can reduce pain from illness or abuse. "Sleep" can put to sleep parts tired from memory work or programmed to harm the body or go to the group. "Forget" can keep memories from the front person so that they can function better or can make a reporter part forget to report. Calling out a particular part by touching the left shoulder and saying that part's name can be used in an emergency. Cooperation is always to be preferred to coercion, so ask or suggest rather than just doing such things.

The following two triggers may be helpful with some survivor clients: Grasping both your client's arms firmly and briefly halfway between the shoulders and elbows will turn off a spinning program temporarily. Holding your hands out in front of you, palms upward, then drawing them quickly towards your chest and closing them will temporarily turn off all programs. If you use these or other triggers (such as special touches or hand signals), make sure that your client's knowledgeable parts have confirmed what effect they will have and agreed to allow you to use them. Also, explain how you learned these triggers. And check with the client that the perpetrators have not changed the meaning of these triggers since reading this book!

When the whole personality system works together, and those insiders in charge work for healing, your client can make substantial recovery, given careful timing and containment, maintaining current physical safety as much as possible, updating the parts about present-day life, encouraging internal communication, doing memory work when the system is ready, and maintaining a good therapeutic relationship.

CHAPTER 7

Present-day physical safety

Therapists working with adult survivors of childhood trauma generally assume that the trauma is long past and that all the survivor is dealing with is residual feelings from what happened long ago. But with victims of ritual abuse and mind control, this is frequently not the case.

The Extreme Abuse Survey results are available at http://eassurvey. wordpress.com/extreme-abuse-survey-final-results/. This survey compared extreme abuse victims who reported ritual abuse (RA) and/or mind control (MC) with those who did not, and this is what they found: The therapist had discovered the survivor was reporting to perpetrators about therapy in 50% of the ritual abuse and/or mind control cases, and 20% of the cases of extreme abuse where ritual abuse and mind control were not reported. The therapist had discovered the abuse was ongoing in 64% of the ritual abuse and/or mind control cases, and 40% of the other extreme abuse cases. And, of course, some of those who did not tell their therapists about ongoing abuse and reporting might not have been consciously aware of it.

Many times, our clients are being abused by the perpetrator groups on an ongoing basis, while we are treating them, and we don't even realize it. Our clients' deliberately designed dissociative disorders keep the knowledge of the ongoing abuse from the parts of the person who attend the therapy sessions. It took me a long time to discover my first such clients were still involved with the perpetrator group, and I missed it with at least one other client.

Assessing a survivor client's safety is difficult. Current abusers have access to the victim's "black book" (which is the abusers' record of the victim's programming) and know which parts to call out with which signals. Front parts are quickly put inside when abuser contact happens, and child parts as well as adult victim parts are brought out by perpetrators for rituals, re-abuse, or retraining. Survivors spend much of their lives in pain. Pain from current events is not recognized as different, since they frequently experience body memories of abuse, usually as punishment for disobedience. They have difficulty telling the difference between current illness, recent injury, and body memories. There is usually extensive programming for the front parts not to remember current events involving the abuser group. "This did not happen." All this makes it difficult to tell when a survivor is still (or again) being abused.

Also, young parts may believe abuse just happened when it didn't, since they haven't been out in the body for many years and don't realize much time has gone by. They live in the past, at the point where their maturing stopped. They may believe perpetrators are around when they are dead and/or gone. They may not understand past versus present, or hallucination versus reality. Young child parts believe the deceptions that were originally used on them as well as new deceptions. They believe the BIG LIE, that the abusers know everything. Survivors are often mistaken about whether they are physically safe. I have seen clients who were being hurt frequently while their front parts were unaware of it, and I have seen clients who were physically safe but believed they were not.

In relation to current safety, therapists make two opposite common mistakes. The first is failing to recognize that current or renewed contact with perpetrators and possible re-abuse is a major concern, and that a client may report anything disclosed in therapy to perpetrators and be punished for disclosures. The second is buying into the survivor's belief (based on the BIG LIE) that perpetrators know everything and are everywhere and all-powerful, and that the client and/or therapist will be killed for talking (though it has to be noted that advancements in cellphone technology have made it less of a lie that the perpetrators know a lot about what is currently going on with the survivor).

Healing goes much faster if your client can establish and maintain physical safety. Perpetrator groups have more manpower hours available than we do to undo any gains our clients make. Perpetrator groups are very bold and aggressive in retraumatizing and threatening survivors who are in therapy. Our objective as therapists with regard to current safety needs to be to help our clients see what is happening to them in the present and make decisions on the basis of that knowledge.

Access programming

Access programming is designed by the perpetrators to put a survivor in immediate contact with the perpetrator group if any disclosures are made about the abuse. It is important to slow down your client's disclosures in the early stages of therapy, reassure them that your purpose is not to make them tell what happened, and work instead on establishing rapport and safety. All survivors have access programming.

Insiders who maintain group contact

- "Returners" have been told to return to the group on significant dates like birthdays, or predetermined ritual dates, or years when the survivor reaches a certain age, or if security has been compromised
- "Reporters" report to perpetrators about disclosures the survivor has made, therapy sessions, and plans to relocate
- Inside parts who "come when called" feel compelled to respond to access triggers through such behaviors as answering the phone, opening the door, leaving the window open, or crossing the street in response to a hand signal.

"Return" programming: training to return to family and/or perpetrators

Some parts have memorized specific dates to "wake up" and return to the group. There are scheduled ritual dates and callback dates.

Often the survivor is supposed to return to the perpetrators if some parts have been disloyal.

The survivor may feel a desperate need to return to the group to:

- Avoid punishment of self or others
- Attend a scheduled ritual or report at a scheduled callback date
- Have a disabling program turned off (be "fixed")
- Find out the facts of what happened
- Save someone else
- Get revenge
- Receive rewards—sex, drugs, or a promotion.

I have seen all these motivations in action. Be alert if your client says they must go home for any one of these reasons. If the survivor does not respond to these programs, the family may devise an "emergency" like an illness for which the front person must return.

If a survivor returns home (to the group) after making disclosures, the reporting parts report disclosures the survivor has made. Punishment is administered for disobedience or disloyalty. Disobedient parts are locked away and replaced in their jobs with backups. Old program training is repeated. Threats are made to the survivor and others: "If you disobey again, a child will be hurt." In some cases, the survivor is drugged and their therapist is impersonated by a group member who assaults the poor survivor verbally, physically, and/or sexually. The survivor may be forced to harm someone else to demonstrate loyalty. The retraining session ends with electroshock to make the survivor forget.

When I was working with my first group of four survivors, I made a rule that current contact memories must be worked through as soon as possible along with the memories of the programs that the current contact attempted to reinstall. That is how I learned about the various programs.

"Report" programming

Watcher and reporter parts observe the survivor's behavior and thoughts, including internal discussions, and report any indications of disloyalty to internal or external bosses. They may be trained to report every word of a conversation to the perpetrators, especially what happens in therapy sessions, and to always tell the truth to perpetrators, who they believe already know everything. Needless to say, they do this out of fear, believing they or their pet or someone they love will be tortured and killed if they stop doing this job. Reporter parts are usually terrified kids who believe the BIG LIE (that the group knows everything—see Chapter 3).

If a survivor discloses secrets, a part who loves family may feel an urge to call home. This part calls (or answers the phone when family calls) and remembers only a normal conversation. The family member is trained to receive these calls, and the front parts of the child believe that family member is innocent. The family member, perhaps a favorite sibling or aunt, calls out a reporter part who tells what is happening in therapy and describes any disloyalty. The family member then calls out other parts and gives them orders, for example, harass the therapist, cut your arms, return home immediately.

Some survivors spend their whole lives moving, trying to get away from abusers without realizing they have parts reporting their location. Relocation is useless until reporting is disabled. I briefly received a high-level cult member client from a therapist in another location and had to smuggle her out of town when she told me that she had reported that she was seeing me. I helped one of my first survivor clients move to a different community. She told me that in my city (Victoria, BC) she could recognize and avoid the abusers, but she didn't recognize the ones who got hold of her in the new place.

The most effective way of dealing with reporting is to speak with the personality system leaders, the ones originally put in charge by the perpetrators. These leaders have not been told about the reporters inside. Inner leaders are supposed to believe the group knows things by magic, science, or surveillance. They likely do not know how the perpetrator group gets hold of them, if it does. They just find themselves called out by the perpetrators and don't know how they got there. These leaders have been told they are in charge of all inside parts. They will be indignant at discovering (from you) that there are reporter parts who are not under their authority.

You can talk to them through the presenting part: "I want your inner leaders to pay attention; I am talking to you, not the front person. You are the key to recovery. You can tell the rest of the system to change their loyalty, to be loyal to your own true self. Why should you do this? ... Because *you* have been deceived by the abusers. The biggest deception is that the abusers know everything you do. They don't. They create reporter parts whom they hide from you. If the abusers knew everything about you, why would they need to create reporter parts to tell them things?" Inner leaders are not little kids and can think this through and see the logic. The inner leaders can order other parts to find the reporters and help them give up their jobs, as they come to understand that reporting causes re-abuse. Of course, you can't speak with the inner leaders early in therapy. It takes time to win their trust. That is why in the early stages of therapy you must try to avoid interventions that will lead to new reporting, or if reported will indicate to abusers that a therapeutic bond has been established or secrets have been divulged.

What do you do if reporter parts are telling perpetrators about therapy sessions? Some reporters may agree to do their jobs by reporting to the inner leaders or to inner copies of the abusers instead of to outside people. It is possible, if reporters won't cooperate, to ask whether the system might be willing to use the "sleep" program on the reporters after the first five minutes of your therapy session and wake them up near the end when you're talking about nothing much. Or system leaders can use the "forget" program to make the reporters forget what happened, substituting a memory of a harmless session. (This is a technique that programmers use to disguise their own interventions.)

If the person must have ongoing telephone contact with family members involved with the abuser group, the inner leaders can make sure the reporters remember nothing that is really reportable. Sometimes reporter parts can learn to lie to abusers so that therapy sessions sound innocuous when the sessions are destroying the programming. This begins with helping them realize that abusers don't know everything; that the BIG LIE is actually a lie. The training to tell the truth to perpetrator group members must also be overcome.

Availability programming

Children are trained to leave the door unlocked or the window open. A survivor may think they feel suffocated if it is closed. They are trained not to run, that running will bring on severe punishment. They are taught not to move or make a noise when being hurt or threatened. Some parts are trained to answer the phone or open the door or go to the handler, afraid for their lives if they don't. The ones who answer the phone may have been punished by someone in a Satan suit who told them, "Always answer when Satan calls." The abusers may simulate car and plane crashes to teach a child that such things will happen if they ever try to move away. Each of these trainings involves severe punishment for noncompliance. Addicted parts are trained to go outside to get their drugs; a message to these parts brings them out, and the survivor feels the symptoms of drug withdrawal.

Monitoring of survivors

When the survivor is no longer returning or reporting, he or she may still be accessible because of parts trained to respond to cues from the perpetrators. These cues are an important means for the perpetrator groups to control adult survivors who are living away from the perpetrator group members. Cards, gifts, emails, or texts from family may contain deliberate triggers to set off programs or give instructions. Specific auditory triggers such as a certain pattern of phone rings, a car honk, beeping sounds, or a pattern of knocks on the door will bring out parts who respond to them. A touch on the left shoulder with the spoken name of a part forces that part out into the body.

Hand and face signals are used to give messages to particular parts in a mind-controlled personality system. They may convey such things as "Come here," "Don't listen to that person," "Tell me if you have misbehaved," or "Turn on the flashbacks." Perpetrator group leaders take leadership positions in churches, online discussion groups, and support groups to gain power and respectability, and to have the opportunity to give signals to many survivors. Many if not most survivors are monitored by people they know. They are permitted to be friends only with other survivors who are forced to report on them. Survivor therapists are sent clients who will report on them.

When survivors are going to be around other survivors, for example at a conference, perpetrators may give some people's inside parts instructions to use hand signals on the other survivors. A survivor may give another survivor a hand signal while the front parts of both people are unaware it is happening. Many hand signals are disguised as ordinary movements. One speaker at a conference I attended was doing this blatantly and was furious when told not to, saying in a tone of ridicule that she was only brushing hair back from her face and adjusting her glasses. She gathered people at the back of the room after her talk in order to continue giving the signals. Cult members also hang around downtowns using hand, foot, or voice signals to find survivors from other groups.

Handlers (minders)

Disobedient survivors of ritual abuse and mind control are likely to be sent handlers—persons who keep contact with them on behalf of the perpetrator group. Often a spouse or an adult child is a handler (sometimes called a minder). Be suspicious of a new boyfriend or a new bosom buddy who appears in a survivor's life suddenly. In addition to the regular handlers, there are traveling programmers who pay visits to survivors to keep them in line. Such people are sent when reporter parts or other victims alert the group that the survivor is making disclosures.

If a survivor is no longer reporting to handlers or family members or attending perpetrator group events, the group escalates their harassment. They will give signals to turn on programs that may give the survivor symptoms that may get the survivor into hospital. Psychiatric hospitals are generally infiltrated, along with many other helping institutions (see Chapter 5). Some symptoms are also designed to discredit a survivor who remembers too much. One of my first survivor clients was diagnosed with paranoid schizophrenia, and I believe his symptoms were designed so that no one would believe the events he remembered and talked about. For example, he had several parts who believed they were celebrities, and when I asked how this came about, he remembered being spun on a turntable surrounded by pictures of celebrities and told to internalize them.

If your client comes from a family with important status in a big multigenerational group, it may be very difficult to achieve physical safety, as the client may be followed and tortured repeatedly. If your client has been publicly disclosing important secrets of the perpetrator group, it may be very difficult for the client to remain safe. Groups are aggressive and bold in harassing survivors; they rely on the survivor's dissociation to keep their harassment from memory, while the terrified parts hold the memories of punishment for disobedience.

Recognizing plants in survivors' lives

If a survivor is trying to get free, it is important that they learn to identify which persons they know may be giving them signals or warnings. They can then be careful not to be alone with such people, or not to reveal anything to them if they must have conversations with them. Those parts of your client who respond to signals can identify and interpret the signals, and if they are cooperative with the healing process, can tell inner leaders immediately when they see or hear such a signal. Your client can learn that if they feel strange or fearful after being in a group of people, they can ask inside to discover who gave them what signals, and what those signals mean.

If a new person appears in your client's life, does it seem a coincidence that the survivor has met this person at this moment? Is the person overly friendly, appearing to have too much in common with the survivor, or flattering them, telling them how wonderful they are? Is the person overly loving, appealing to little ones who were not loved? Does the person seem to know too much about ritual abuse, mind control, abuser networks, and/or dissociative disorders? Does the person show signs of dissociation such as too much forgetfulness and unexpected rudeness? Do they demonstrate the kind of entitled, demanding, or demeaning behavior typical of perpetrators? Do they suddenly appear in your client's life, showing a lot of interest in them, then disappear, then reappear? And, of course, do they use any hand, face, or touch signals that might set off programs? Any of these things might indicate that they have been sent by the perpetrator group.

Perpetrators who present themselves as helpers can fool a therapist, too. A leader of a helping organization, a therapist, or another other health service provider can be a plant. In addition to the criteria described above, does such a person seem to lack compassion and act from just intellect? Or fake compassion and warmth? Does the person seem to know too little about areas in which they claim expertise? Are they rigidly attached to one approach, speaking as if reciting without tolerating interruption? Do they twist the truth about other people, accusing possibly innocent people of being perpetrators or plants?

Some safety precautions for survivors

If there's current danger, your client might consider trying to have a safe partner or roommate who can be informed and stay with them whenever they go out but is kind enough to give them "alone time" when they need it. But it is important to be absolutely sure the supposedly safe person is uninvolved with the perpetrators, as well as brave enough to knowingly enter into this situation.

It is important that the survivor make sure no programs on their phone are recording conversations. They can turn off the phone ringer so no part will respond immediately to a call. They can erase text messages without reading them. They can leave their cellphone in the fridge or remove its battery so it can't be tracked when they go out. They can change their email address. (This will, of course, only be helpful if no part reports the change to the perpetrators.) If they know that letters and parcels are likely to trigger programming, they can decide to open them only in the therapy office, where they can discuss the meaning of any triggers. Most importantly, when they are ready, they should work through the memories of the access trainings so that the parts involved no longer feel the urge to do their jobs.

How the groups try to kill survivors

The groups do kill survivors who are disclosing too much and seriously endangering the security of the perpetrator group. The preferred method is to make homicide look like suicide. Overdosing a victim with his or her own pills. Putting cyanide pills on top of someone's usual pills. Slitting a drugged survivor's wrists. Two of my first survivor clients had cult members break into their homes, find their pills, and shove all of them down their throats. Even acetaminophen (Tylenol) is lethal if you ingest a whole bottle. In Chapter 1 of *Healing the Unimaginable*, I told the story of Lorraine, another of my first survivor clients, whose apparent suicide I believe was murder.

The groups can also tamper with a survivor's (or a therapist's) car. I had a brake cable snap twice within a year. They can have a suicide soldier drive into someone's car. They can push someone off a bridge. They can order someone to jump off a building, which a part of a victim might do to save someone else's life. They can slip poison into someone's food, especially at events. Some victims are trained to do that. I believe it is now rare for such groups to try to kill therapists. Still, it can be useful for us and our survivor clients to make a list of present-day perpetrators and leave it with safe people. When perpetrators know there is such a list, they may think twice.

Bas Kremer of the Netherlands wrote on the Organized and Extreme Abuse discussion list of the International Society for the Study of Trauma and Dissociation: "We are dealing not only with the most serious crime imaginable, but also with networks that over generations have refined how to protect themselves."

Guidelines about clients' and your own safety

To summarize my guidelines about the issue of present-day physical safety for survivor clients: Be aware that many if not most survivors of ritual abuse and mind control are still involved with perpetrators and will report to them any disclosures they make. Be aware that pressing for memories too soon will trigger this. The work is much easier if they are not reporting. Look for signs of ongoing abuse and group involvement. Recognize that your client's front person probably does not know whether they are safe. It is not up to you to keep them physically safe. You should, however, make it a priority for them to gain awareness of present intimidation so they can make intelligent decisions. Recognize that your client may be re-abused and tortured regularly, but it is their decision whether to continue in therapy once they are aware of this.

Talk through to your client's inner parts, and ask them to be sure to inform you if they are currently being hurt, even if the abusers are threatening your life. Say that you knew of the risk when you took on this work, and you will be safer if the current abusers know that you know about them.

CHAPTER 8

Working through the traumatic memories

Perpetrator groups are afraid of their victims' programming being undone and of their secret, evil practices being discovered. As both these things happen when their victims put their memories together, the groups are determined to prevent survivors looking at their memories. That is the reason for the constant harassment of survivors. But full healing for survivors can only come about when they put together their training memories.

The importance of having a witness

Full acknowledgment of abuse can only truly take place when the survivor has a witness, someone who will listen to them with compassion and the willingness to believe. Otherwise, the survivor can easily discount the severity and importance of their experiences. Do not underestimate the power of witnessing. I know that someone else's acknowledgment of my own experience of interpersonal trauma, including resonating with my feelings about it, has been very healing. So, whatever method of memory processing you and your client use, just remember that the therapeutic relationship is primary, not the technical methodology. During the witnessing, as a survivor goes through a traumatic memory, it is important that the witness respond appropriately, with compassion and curiosity, asking questions, completely tuned in to the survivor. When there is no external witness, there can be internal witnesses, other parts of a survivor who listen to the stories of the other traumatized parts.

Three phases of treatment

The ISST-D guidelines recommend three phases of treatment:

1) Establishing safety, stabilization, and symptom reduction
2) Confronting, working through, and integrating traumatic memories, and
3) Integration and rehabilitation.

Many survivors of mind-controlling abuses never get beyond Phase 1 because there is so much built in to their personality systems to prevent the actual traumatic memories from surfacing, in particular the memories of the foundation building and programming. However, if a survivor doesn't work through the traumatic memories, they will remain fragmented and constantly fighting against impulses or feelings coming from these experiences. Genuine integration of most parts will not occur, though they may learn to cooperate internally.

Deciding whether and when to pursue memories

If a survivor tries to work with memories too early in the recovery process, the security system will be triggered and parts will do jobs such as punishing the person for disobedience and reporting to perpetrators. It is wise for a survivor not to do memory work until internal leaders agree to it or at least agree to certain relatively innocuous memories being worked on. It may also be wise for a survivor not to do memory work during periods of current life stress, as it can cause bodily and emotional symptoms when memories are only partially processed, and these will interfere with the survivor's day to day functioning. It is also unwise to work on several memories at once, as emotions may flood and memories may remain incomplete.

But if the survivor wants to be free of programming, free of unpleasant and disabling symptoms, and able to choose their own life path, memory work is essential. When you have a good therapeutic relationship, including establishing some trust with the higher-up parts, you and your client can make a joint decision to pursue memory work. The most effective method of freeing survivors from the mind control, fears, and behavioral compulsions ("jobs") assigned to parts is working through the memories of the training that created the mind control.

Delay memory work until the client is ready, but at a certain point, you can tell that those in charge of the system are letting some memories, or parts of memories, that are ready to be dealt with come out. You have the cooperation of system leaders, and internal punishment for disclosure is likely to be light. Then it is time to proceed cautiously with memory processing.

Dealing with flashbacks

The fact that memories (usually flashbacks of parts of memories) come up does not indicate the survivor is ready to work them through. A flashback is a memory fragment, a "closed physiological loop of re-abuse," which can be visual (hallucinations), auditory (voices, noises, screams), emotional (panic, despair, shame), or physiological ("body memory," for example of rape or drugs or shock). With mind control or ritual abuse survivors, most flashbacks are deliberately sent as punishment. Instead of pursuing the memories that flash back, it is wisest for the survivor to ask internally that those in charge of the internal memory files put the flashbacks away and instead choose memories to process strategically. Not every memory needs to be worked through immediately, although it is helpful to keep a record of it so that it can be approached later.

For flashbacks in the therapy session, you can help your survivor client to use grounding. For example, you can ask the client to open their eyes, find and name five things they can see, four things they can feel, three things they can hear, two things they can smell, and one thing they can taste. The survivor can also touch their clothes, which reassures them that their clothes are on their body, place their feet on the ground, touch the arms of the chair they are sitting in, and wiggle their toes inside their shoes and feel the sensation.

It is helpful to establish a signal that you can use to bring your client back to the present if they are caught in a flashback experience, such as placing your right hand on their right shoulder while saying the word "Stop!" (Never use the left hand on the left shoulder, because this is used by abuser groups to call out parts to do their bidding. It is painful to the victim and this pain will be felt if you do this.) It is also helpful to teach your client to use grounding if a flashback happens when they are alone.

If you know program "off" triggers and the client is aware of how you came to know them, you can use them (if you have the client's permission ahead of time) to turn off the program causing the flashback. It is most important to teach your client internal negotiation (with the parts *causing* the flashback, not the ones *experiencing* it), so that flashbacks can be reduced. They are usually punishment for some behavior judged unacceptable by the abusers, so that can be made explicit in the internal dialogue (or dialogue with you), and decisions can be made by the system about whether that behavior needs to change.

Planning memory work

The ISST-D Treatment Guidelines have some helpful advice:

> It is optimal to carefully plan out and schedule work on traumatic memories. Patient and therapist should discuss and reach agreement upon which memories will be the focus, at what level of intensity they will be processed, which types of interventions may be used (i.e., exposure, planned abreactions, etc.), which alternate identities will participate, what steps will be taken to maintain safety during the work, and which procedures will be used to contain traumatic memories if the work becomes too intense. Patients benefit when therapists help them use planning and exploratory and titration strategies … to develop a sense of control over the emergence of traumatic material. … In this phase, as the various elements of a traumatic memory emerge,

they are generally explored rather than redissociated or rapidly contained—assuming that there is adequate time in sessions and that the patient can do this work without significant life disruptions.

As topics come up in therapy, you and/or your survivor client should keep a record of groups of parts (insiders) who need memory work, or of memories (or programs) that need to be dealt with, as well as a transcript of the memory work sessions. Full memory work sessions should preferably be at least ninety minutes long.

Booby traps regarding memory work

As you plan your memory work, you can ask, "What will happen if we try to undo this particular [suicide/pain/report/open door] program?" Memories of training sessions may be linked, so that if you work on one program, another program is turned on. If so, get a "wiring diagram." The client who taught me about this said that if she tried to put together the memory that caused her to flood with unwanted emotions, it would trigger the program that made her believe she was a perpetrator. If she tried to put this memory together, it would trigger a suicide program. It was current abusers who had created these linkages. She learned to put these connections into a diagram to find out which memories were relatively safe to approach, with consequences we could deal with, such as turning on a program that she had already dismantled and could no longer be turned on.

Choosing memories to work with

Begin with relatively easy traumatic memories, minor traumas without too much shock or horror or physical pain, memories that are not part of the basic training (programming). Working through these more accessible memories allows the survivor to learn the process. The system leaders may be aware of some such events and permit work on them. As you help your client do this work, they and other parts can observe and see how it resolves the trauma of those parts involved in these memories.

With "regular" abuse survivors, a therapist usually waits for the memories to emerge and works with those that are emerging. Mind control survivors, however, will be wiser to choose the memories strategically from the internal files to dismantle the programming, beginning with programs that compromise the survivor's safety. You can discuss the strategy with your client.

Once a suitable processing method is established and agreed on, and the system leaders are on board, it is time to have the system choose memories on a logical basis, with the goal being safety. Suicide and self-harm and access programs (including reporting training) are priorities. Eventually, once most programming has been worked through, you can work chronologically to clean up unprocessed memories. Don't forget the infant memories of the original splits. Infant memories are accessible with survivors of deliberate early splitting in a way that they are not with the rest of us. Slightly older parts can translate the infant parts' experiences into words, or recite the words the baby heard, even if the baby didn't understand them.

These abuser groups organize personality systems with storage systems for memories and files that record all trainings, when and where they happened and for what purpose, how often each type of training was repeated, and which parts of the person were trained. They do this so they can keep track of survivors' programmed skills and reestablish trained behaviors when they deem it necessary. A survivor can search their internal files (held by librarians or file keepers) for the necessary information. The internal record may list everything a survivor needs to know—which parts (insiders) are in a memory, when the event occurred, what it was training for, etc. However, if a victim has been especially rebellious, different bits of related information and internal parts from the same memory may be stored in different sections of the personality system. Nevertheless, a victim is one human being, and when that person is determined to recover and to work through the memories, their brain will respond by finding what they need to know. Program codes held by internal programmers can provide information about how many times a particular training was done, at what ages and where. It is rare that an important "lesson" is taught only once.

You and your client's front parts do not need to know what the memory the client is going to process contains before you begin. Just something like "the memory that makes you cut your arms," or "the memory that makes you leave your window open." I rarely knew anything about what a memory would contain when I began it with a client, and neither did the client's front parts. I liked it this way, as I could not be accused of suggesting anything to the client.

Memory components

It is important to realize that very early in a child's life, mind-controlling abusers separate off particular emotions and bodily sensations into different internal "people." For that reason, you can't assume that when your client puts their story together, all these aspects of the memory will naturally come up. Abusers frequently deliberately hide physical and emotional pain holder parts to prevent memories from being thoroughly worked through. They then use the dissociated pain as punishment for the victim trying to achieve freedom.

Processing a memory must include all aspects of what happened. Getting the story is not sufficient. If a survivor gets the full narrative (sight and sound content) of the memory without the feelings, it may make it easier for the person (front parts) to be aware of the deceptions and work hard to resist mind-controlled behaviors. But there is a risk of the emotions belonging to the memory flooding the survivor because a partially completed memory struggles to complete itself, and the emotions and body sensations may be overwhelming. Also, without the emotions worked through in conjunction with the narrative, the "rational" parts of the person may continue to be unaware of the evil of what happened, and parts may still feel compelled to do their "jobs" for the abusers.

In everyday life, we who are not dissociative are generally unaware of the complexity of what we are experiencing with our senses. Every experience includes sight, hearing, smell, taste, and bodily sensations, which include the softness or hardness or spikiness of what we touch or what touches us, itches, pain (which may be dull, sharp, prolonged, or brief), sexual feelings, drugged sensations, and sensations of motion, balance, and dizziness. Electroshock is an important component of many training memories. All these components of experience must be put together when a trauma survivor processes the memory of the trauma.

Every experience also involves emotions, and traumatic experiences usually involve intense, often unbearable, emotions. The worst are despair, sorrow, terror, fury, and shame. As with physical pain, emotional pain is frequently segmented into particular inside parts or "people."

Parts who must be included in memory work

A trauma is not resolved until all aspects of it have been joined: knowledge, sight, hearing, touch, and taste, pain, drugs, and each emotion involved. A memory usually involves several insider parts of the person (inner people), each of whom holds a particular feeling, sensation, or piece of knowledge. Working through a memory thoroughly (especially including all sensory and emotional components) puts together the entire story of the memory, dissolves the strong emotions and impulses coming from that memory, and integrates parts of the person. Organized abuser groups know this and put in programming to prevent memories being fully reconstituted. Reactivator parts are trained to take and withhold specific parts of important training memories.

Reactivator parts (see Chapter 4) are trained to deliberately withhold and hide a small part of each training memory, so that the training effect (program) cannot be destroyed and the perpetrator group can recreate the damaged program from the missing piece. Reactivator parts, like reporters, are hidden from the inner leaders. It is important before you process memories to look for reactivator parts. Ask whether anyone inside has the job of keeping pieces of the memories separate. Enter into dialogue with these parts and make sure their piece is included every time you process a memory. If their part is put into the memory, it is much more difficult for the perpetrator group to reestablish the program. One of my first survivor clients made tremendous progress in processing her training memories and preventing her programs from working. But I didn't yet know about reactivator parts. The cult made a plan to kill off all my clients at once. Right after one of them was murdered (disguised as suicide, see Chapter 1 of *Healing the Unimaginable*), the cult set off programs in the remaining ones. The young woman who had made such progress suddenly discovered that all her programs were working again and turned on, creating havoc in her personality system and putting her at risk. She had to go through all the memories we had processed together and add in the reactivators' pieces in order to permanently disable the programs.

Many if not most organized personality systems include traumatized infants with strong emotions, trapped in boxes or other storage units of highly protected sections of the brain. These parts have been hidden so that the person will not show any emotions, and those emotions can be used to power suicide and other programs. It is important for the survivor to find those infants, set them free, and include them in memory processing.

All training events split off parts to carry the training and usually create backups for the parts who are supposed to engage in the trained behaviors. Backups must be included in memory work.

Sophisticated programming groups call out sets of parts belonging to a particular training and order some of those parts to go somewhere else in the inner landscape, so that they will be omitted from memory work. Find them.

Front people and memories

I have observed that if the parts involved in a particular memory have released their feelings in relation to the memory, the programming will be resolved and the whole person will feel better, and eventually the knowledge will come to the front people when more of the trauma has been worked through. Front people have a lot to deal with in present-day life and may fail to manage their life if major traumatic memories are revealed to them too early. They will have their own emotional reaction to the knowledge. Remember that the front people are no more "real" than the insiders.

However, whether the front parts take part in the memory processing is a decision for the survivor's system. Every system is different. Some survivors have very strong front people who want to be involved in all memory work and can handle it. Many do not. As the therapist, be careful about giving your opinion about such questions. Survivors are very sensitive to being told what to do and may take an opinion of yours as an order when it is not meant that way.

Recording memory work

At the time a memory is processed, it is as if it is experienced for the first time. It remains distinct and has not been blended with other similar memories because its components have been kept separate from one another and from other memories. Once it has been fully processed, however, its details can become less distinct in memory. Because of this, it is important to keep a clear record of what was said during the memory processing. My practice was to write down everything a client said during the memory processing, as they spoke it, so they could discuss it with me later. Writing out verbatim what the client has said provides a much more accurate summary of what has gone on than the brief notes that many therapists write after a session is over. I could never remember much about a session after it ended because I was concentrating too much on the process and on my attunement to the client rather than focusing on the details of the content. I suspect most therapists are like me in this regard. My detailed record of memory work sessions was helpful when new parts were found who were involved in the same kind of training as some we had worked with. We could revisit the memory we had worked on and add what the newly found parts held. Adding pieces to a memory doesn't usually take long.

It is also important to keep a record of all memories worked with and their purpose if they are training memories. Basic training (programming) is conducted repeatedly for each important program, for example at ages three, six, and nine. Internal programmers may have codes that tell you when and where each training was done. As your client becomes proficient at memory work, they may be able to combine all the repetitions of a particular training into one memory work session, just acknowledging the differences in the details.

Confidential clinical records should be stored very securely, as abusers want to see what has gone on in therapy. One of my first clients, seen at the mental health center where confidential files of all therapists were kept in a central location, brought me what she said were her "programs." They turned out to be photocopies of my notes about another client's programs! Needless to say, I stopped using the central storage system for my own confidential files. Abuser groups place members strategically in such positions as secretary in an office and ward clerk in a psychiatric hospital.

Processing a memory

Beginning the memory processing

The survivor should gather all inner people (parts) who have any part of the particular memory to be processed in a safe internal place with a way of viewing and hearing the memories. Clients who were used for pornographic films might have trouble with video, so it is important that the survivor choose the way to see the memory. The survivor may now choose a narrator part to tell the story as it proceeds during the video. Prepare to take notes or tape the narration, as this is the best record of the trauma and training, as the memory details will fade once the memory is consciously known and its emotional charge removed.

Similar memories can sometimes be processed together. For example, if a training was repeated at ages three, six, and nine, your client can process these events together and then add the incidental details that were different. The parts involved in each of the three trainings all need to be present.

Feelings in memory processing

Survivors of childhood trauma often have great difficulty distinguishing between feelings or sensations that belong to memories, feelings that belong to recent trauma, and feelings that are indicators of illness. It is important that they find insider parts who can tell the difference, because present-day illness and recent injury must be dealt with. Recent injury can come from harassment from perpetrators. Too often survivors neglect actual illness or injury because they assume it is a chronic condition or just "memory pain." So, when strong emotions or bodily sensations come up for your client, help them problem-solve about the source.

The way a traumatic memory spontaneously comes up is often with the experience of an emotional state and bodily sensations, before the story of what caused these feelings emerges. Programmers use these separated dissociated emotions as punishment for disobedient victims.

The feelings only come to make sense once the story of the memory is put together. If a survivor is used to accessing memories in this way, feelings first, they may expect to continue doing this. It is the feelings (both physical sensations, such as pain and spinning, and strong emotions) that can become overwhelming as a survivor approaches a traumatic memory and can make the process get stuck. Spinning at the end of deliberately designed traumas is designed to have this effect.

Because of this, my preferred method for memory work involves deliberately separating out the feelings (both physical and emotional) while putting together the story, then adding in the feelings once the story is known. I refined this from the method I learned in a workshop by Judith Peterson around 1993. Many survivors of organized abuse are able to do this because their structured dissociation has already separated feelings to be held by particular parts of the person.

If you and your client choose this method, the survivor needs to create in their inner world a place where unprocessed memories and feelings are to be kept in containers, as well as some containers. One survivor may use an (imaginary) cave with barrels, another may use a bank vault with storage lockers, and another may use a storage room with jars on shelves. There should also be a place for partially processed memories (left unfinished between memory work sessions). Containers should have a way to add to them without the contents spilling out (a spout, a straw, a door), as it is common that feelings will come up and create a problem during the memory processing, and they will need to be deliberately separated out.

Dissociating the feelings

You, or an inner leader, will now guide the gathered insiders to put feelings into the container, naming feelings, such as pain, dizziness, drugged sensations, sexual feelings, emotions like fear, worry, anger, sadness, and hopelessness, and anything else that was felt in any part of the body, or any other emotions that belong to this memory. Make sure that inner people are not put into the container, even if they have previously held some of these feelings. When all the feelings are inside, the survivor can lock up the container.

Processing the story of a memory

Now, the survivor uses the internal filing system to access "videos" or "files" of memories. (The way the memories are stored depends on the age of the survivor and what methods were used during their childhood training.) All insiders holding any parts of the memory observe the memory event (sight and sound only) while the feelings remain in the container. The client (usually a specific internal part who is assigned this job) holds the remote control and can make the picture and sound bigger or smaller, speed it up or slow it down, rewind, fast forward, pause, or stop. Any of these things can be used to make the process easier or clearer. The narrator, who is "out" in the body, tells or writes down what they are seeing and hearing. If sound is not mentioned, ask for it. Sound is often omitted, and is important, as the programming instructions are in the words used by the perpetrators.

If a client is processing a memory in my office, I interact constantly with the client, asking clarification questions, giving reassurances that it is not happening now, and correcting cognitive distortions as they happen, pointing out lies and tricks as they are observed. So, the whole process is a dialogue about a visual and auditory narrative. Go through the story from apparent safety (ordinary life) through trauma to safety again. There are often front parts present at the beginning and again at the end. If the memory is too long to process in one session, your client may need to place it in temporary storage in a labeled internal container and return to it in subsequent sessions. If the client is sufficiently skilled, they can work on it alone.

Integrating the feelings

If the emotions and the bodily sensations are not processed, the entire memory can easily be re-dissociated, pain-holder parts remain stuck in that experience, flashbacks may occur, and programming is not destroyed. So, you can't just leave the feelings in the container for very long. Take a breather in the real world after the story has been told. The survivor can even lock up the memory and process the feelings in the next session. Leaving all the work that has been done in the container will help keep it together until the memory is fully put together.

Once the story is complete and all involved parts know it, the survivor should go through the story again with feelings, either once very slowly or several times, adding more feelings each time. I've had clients who managed the process by doing it once very slowly. I would read aloud the transcript of what the narrator said, and as I said each phrase, the gathered parts briefly experienced the feelings associated with that phrase. Other clients would go through the entire memory, adding in the despair, then again, adding in the fear, then again, adding in the pain, etc. The feelings and physical sensations do not have to be experienced for the duration for which they were originally felt, but they do have to be acknowledged and incorporated into the memory with the story (pictures and sound). When all the feelings have been felt, the survivor can put the whole memory into the container and store it (labeled) in a new internal place for completed memories. Some survivors need to allow the feelings to be felt and released gradually over a period of days after the content processing. It is important for your client to find what works best for them. Each decision a survivor gets to make strengthens their sense of their own power over their lives, something they have been denied since infancy. It is, however, important that you be with the client, resonating with the emotions the person experienced as the horrific event proceeded. The therapeutic relationship is primary.

Your client might like to end the process with a symbolic cleansing in light or water (I prefer a warm, breathable waterfall) where all insiders who took part in the memory are cleansed, inside and out, from any dirty or contaminated feelings, and any remnants of the memory are washed away. I like to say that the waterfall (or light) will wash away any boundaries between inside people who no longer need to be separate and will strengthen boundaries if they need to stay separate, because this is what happens when a memory is processed thoroughly. Before you do it, check with the client about whether the use of any specific method (waterfall, light) would trigger some problematic experience. The perpetrator groups read our books and hear our presentations and put in programming to derail some of the interventions we have developed.

After memory work, have at least one discussion or writing session in which the survivor can deal with their current reactions to what happened, including guilt, shame, horror, and possible integrations of parts. If the front parts need to be unaware of this, you can still engage in this process with insiders.

Resolving traumas through memory processing

A memory that fragmented a person can be reconstituted if it is relived while the person knows they are in a safe place with a safe person. Or completely alone. The fragments of experience belonging to the different senses and emotions are brought together and become integrated. In this way, the memory fragments move from the unconscious to the conscious mind. What was formerly a dissociated, "forgotten" memory is now consciously remembered. It no longer erupts in disturbing ways. It loses much of its emotional punch. When a traumatic memory is put together, some dissociative barriers are no longer necessary, and parts of the person involved in that event often join together. The survivor comes to see clearly how the event was the source of programmed behaviors, and programming that operates like a posthypnotic suggestion is dissolved.

The ISST-D Treatment Guidelines put it this way:

> Integrating traumatic memories involves bringing together aspects of traumatic experience that have been previously dissociated from one another: memories and the sequence of events, the associated affects, and the physiological and somatic representations of the experience. Integration also means that the patient achieves an adult cognitive awareness of his or her role and that of others in the events. Work on loss, grief and mourning may be profound in this stage as the patient grapples with the realization of the many losses that the traumatic past has caused ... The process of Phase 2 work allows the patient to realize that the traumatic experiences belong to the past, to understand their impact in his or her life, and to develop a more complete and coherent personal history and sense of self ... As traumatic experiences are integrated, the alternate

identities may experience themselves as less and less separate and distinct … Over time, and often with repeated iterations, the material in these memories is transformed from traumatic memory into what is generally termed narrative memory … A major mechanism of change is one of repeatedly re-accessing and re-associating and thus integrating fragmented and dissoci- ated elements of traumatic memories into a comprehensible and coherent narrative. (www.isst-d.org)

I have not found it necessary to repeat the same piece of memory work over and over again. The key is to make sure that all internal persons who had part of the memory take part when the memory is processed. However, it is necessary and important to troubleshoot when some- thing appears to be stuck or go wrong during a piece of memory work, and also to discuss the implications of each memory with the client. Discoveries arising from memory work may alter the survivor's life decisions.

This discussion should include the front people if they are aware of the memory but not if they remain amnestic for it. Quite often the front parts do not know what has happened during a therapy session, whether or not it involves memory work, and this is not generally upsetting to them. I have found that memories that are fully processed become known to the front people when they are ready.

Troubleshooting

Troubleshooting during memory work

- Keep monitoring your client's emotional state during the memory work. If feelings become overwhelming, pause the process and remind the insiders to put them into the container.
- If the memory is confused, get the drugged or spinning feelings into the container. Drugs and spinning confuse the child at the time of the abuse, but there are always some parts who know what is going on.
- If the chronological order of the experience is confused, have someone inside line up the insiders in the order in which their pieces come.

- Check for discontinuities that might indicate a missing piece of the memory. It is easy to miss a segment because some insider who has that segment is missing. Survivors often avoid embarrassing parts of memories like sexual feelings, shameful ones like perpetration, or extreme pain.
- If the story gets stuck, take a break to talk with the parts and find out why it is stuck. Look for missing insiders, especially censoring ones regarding sex or shame. Search for the parts of the survivor who hold the missing pieces and help them contribute to the completion of the memory.
- The "soundtrack" involving instructions is very important for the survivor to know in order to destroy programming. Make sure none of it is omitted.

Troubleshooting after memory work

- If the program that this memory created is still working, either a piece of the memory has been omitted or there are other training memories related to the same program.
- Make sure the recyclers have put their pieces in.
- Look for "incidental training," accidental events (such as sounds from outside) that were incorporated into the training session.
- Is the survivor experiencing physical symptoms such as pain afterward? This may indicate that these need to be put together with the part of the memory in which they happened, or that the survivor has been punished (internally or externally) for doing the memory work.
- If the survivor is experiencing emotional symptoms, help them understand whether these belong to the event itself or to a present-day reaction to what has been discovered in this memory. Insiders who became aware of this traumatic event may have their own emotional reactions to discovering what happened, and they need a listening ear.

Teach your client to do their own memory work

Memory work can take a huge number of therapy sessions. Every ritual abuse/mind control/organized abuse survivor has experienced thousands of traumas, especially in childhood. Following the guidelines in this book, memory work can be done in therapy sessions. But it empowers a survivor to be able to work through many of the traumatic and training memories without the therapist present. This is more convenient for the survivor and relieves the pressure on the therapist to do memory work in every session. It shortens the healing process. Every part has a story to tell and needs a witness to that story. Internal witnesses are most important, because they will always be there. An infant can convey a story to child parts a little older who will understand. Internal nurturers can comfort hurt parts as well as listen to them. When your client leaves therapy, they can continue the healing process through internal witnessing and nurturing.

Specific recommendations for mind control survivors

I recommend following the ISST-D Treatment Guidelines, plus certain things that are specifically geared towards ritual abuse and mind control survivors:

1) Planning ahead to choose memories that will unravel programming.
2) Making sure to include all parts of the system, including infants, who hold any part of the memory being processed.
3) Including reactivator parts.
4) Accessing internal files regarding training memories.
5) Temporarily dissociating physical and emotional feelings to get a clear narrative, then integrating those feelings with the memory. This is not essential, but it helps get around the spinning barrier or spinning and electroshock by which many training memories are protected by the perpetrators.

CHAPTER 9

Confronting the spiritual issues in ritual abuse

People have always been trying to understand the world. When bad things happened, we searched for an explanation. We wanted the world to be just and fair. Many primitive societies believed that if bad things happen to people, those people must deserve it. Natural disasters are called "acts of God" by those who don't understand what causes them. Ancient people imagined the gods, good or bad, as causing things, because science hadn't yet been invented. Modern people recognize the external forces that cause problems, such as bacteria, viruses, or faults in the earth's crust, all discovered by science.

Many primitive peoples believed that if a disaster happened, it must be a divine punishment for something bad someone did. The biblical story of Jonah illustrates this belief. Some religions imagined "devils" or "demons" that caused illnesses. Before the discovery of bacteria and viruses, it was widely believed that someone could curse someone else and make them sick. We use the term "bad" for something or someone evil, and also for something unfortunate. It is easy, especially for children, to confuse unfortunate with evil.

Because disasters don't kill everyone, some think that it is God who saves some people from disasters and lets others die; He chooses the good people to save. I cannot accept this belief, because if you thank God for saving you from a disaster that killed some people, you are really thanking Him for killing all those other people.

The Wikipedia entries about Lucifer and "Devil in Christianity" trace the history of belief in those mythical beings. Dante's *Inferno* and Milton's epic poem *Paradise Lost* in the Middle Ages had a major role in developing that mythology. Occult groups, along with fundamentalist Christians, have adopted Milton's story as if it were true. Some believe Satan and Lucifer are the same; others believe that they are two different beings vying for power and take the side of one or the other. So, there are Satanists and Luciferians. Both kinds of groups, as well as many Christian denominations, teach little children about Satan and Lucifer, and the demons they supposedly oversee. Victims of abuse by Satanists know him as the terrifying man in the skintight red suit with horns and a tail.

Simulated religious scenarios

Perpetrator groups infuse their religious ideology into children by putting those children through literal physical experiences. Some of them may do it cynically because children having these beliefs are easier to manipulate. Others may do it because they have the beliefs themselves and believe they are teaching the children the truth. As many perpetrators are themselves victims and therefore dissociative, they may have both approaches within one person. Whatever the motivation, what they do is brutal.

Satan, Lucifer, demons, and hell

The following are experiences which victims report to therapists:

- Hell is simulated for various rituals. There is fire and smoke (made with "dry ice"). Satan appears out of the fire. A victim may also encounter other Satanic beings such as Beelzebub, Satan's messenger, the Beast, and Lucifer. All, of course, are men (and occasionally women) in costumes and masks. They are likely to rape and otherwise harm the child victim. In "hell", people are being visibly tortured, and victims may be given a choice between torturing someone else and being tortured.

- A child is put in a coffin, drugged, falls asleep, and wakes up in "hell." The child is told it is now dead and in hell because it is so evil.
- The "Satanic baptism" and "marriage to Satan" (see Chapter 3), both involving painful rapes of a child by the man in the red Satan suit, are performed in "hell."
- "Demon" parts (see Chapter 4) are "created" (split off) in "hell" through abuse by costumed adults (dressed as big demons). The big demons train the "demon" children on how to behave like demons.
- A child may be made to sign a false contract giving his or her soul to Satan or Lucifer.

God and Jesus

Abuser groups don't stop with their own deities; they also simulate the Christian deities God and Jesus, as well as angels. The following acts have been reported by survivors:

- A child is brought before an older, white-bearded man dressed in a robe, like the familiar depictions of God in Christian art. The child is judged by "God" to be evil. The man verbally abuses the child, an act of utter rejection, saying the child must spend eternity in hell. He may rape the child.
- The child is brought to a younger man who is dressed to look like the traditional pictures of Jesus. The simulated Jesus may turn his back on the child, rape the child, or spit on the child. The child may have to hurt him while "Jesus" is tied to a cross.
- The child may be tied to the cross and tortured by "Jesus."
- A child's hands may be used to kill what is said to be the "baby Jesus."
- A child part is split off and told he is God, Almighty God, or Jesus. This part is taught what to say to the other parts of the victim. It is usually words of rejection but could also be directions ("divine guidance") for behavior, such as suicide.
- The abuser groups simulate angels for their own purposes, particularly the angel of suicide, also called the "angel of mercy" or "angel of the sunset" (see Chapter 3).

Other religious scenarios

Some groups simulate ancient Egyptian and other deities. Like "God" and "Jesus," they can be internalized, given instructions, and used to terrorize the survivor. In other groups, new age beliefs are used instead of Christian ones, with internal voices representing God or spiritual guides, and "spiritual" messages giving directions that benefit the perpetrator group. Inside parts of the survivor are given the job of speaking the "voice of the gods" to the other parts. Such programs as this are always being updated to reflect the beliefs of contemporary culture.

God doesn't rescue

The abuser groups teach children that God won't rescue them. The abusers torture a child and tell that child to pray to God or Jesus to be rescued. The child prays and nothing happens; the torture continues. The abusers suggest praying to Satan instead, then the man in the red suit shows up and the torture stops. Now this child part of the survivor believes he or she is too evil for God's help, and only Satan will help.

It is a reality that God doesn't rescue little children being abused, and whatever our belief system, we need to recognize this reality.

Spiritual/moral abuse: making victims believe they are evil

Attempting to obtain children's lifelong loyalty, the abuser groups work hard to make children believe themselves to be evil. Simulated surgeries put a "black heart" or "Satan's brain" inside a little child, followed by an event to make the child think she or he is now evil because of the black heart or evil brain. Children are drugged to unconsciousness, then dressed up as demons or monsters or aliens. They wake up in costume, and people act as if they are evil and frightening. Parts of a child are trained as psychic killers (witches): they are told to kill a person or animal with their minds, then see that person or animal apparently dying.

Abusers give a child a hallucinogenic drug, then place that child in a triangle inside a pentagram. They tell the child to invite a demon to reside in them. They then torture the child until a new part is split off. This is timed for the moment the drug will take effect. Everyone hails the new part as a demon and pretends to be afraid of it. The child feels weird and disoriented and figures it must really be a demon.

Children are expected and trained to perpetrate acts against other people and animals. In ritually abusive groups, every child has to participate in human and animal sacrifices. The man behind the child tells the child to kill the animal or human victim. The group wants the child to do it without being physically forced, and they keep giving the child forced choices: "You kill this animal, or we kill this child," "Kill the person quickly or we kill them slowly and painfully," "If you won't do it, we will skin the animal alive." Forced killing is often an act of mercy. If the child persists in refusing to cooperate (and various parts are split off in the process), the man uses the child's hand to do the act, with his own stronger hand around it.

Children take part in the black mass, which involves eating human flesh and drinking blood, usually of a sacrificed victim. They must kill (with adult help) a "disposable" friend they have been given, at around age six. A girl is made pregnant at age eleven to thirteen, and she has to use a knife to sacrifice her first baby, said to be "Satan's child." Teen girls are made to give birth to babies who are sacrificed or kept hidden and repeatedly abused. Adult victims are taught to hold a pillow over their babies' faces until they stop crying, to teach them not to cry. And they are made to sexually abuse their own children, believing that those children will be killed if they don't do this. All these events can violate the person's own spirituality and capacity for empathy, splitting off parts who don't or can't feel empathy, and causing an enormous load of shame to be stored within the survivor. Yet some victims sacrifice themselves to save an infant, sometimes not even their own infant.

Certain parts of a child are trained to dissect sacrifices, take out the heart, etc. And some are trained to kill. Some parts are taught to rape (girls use objects). I remember my shock when I discovered how Spiker, a part of my first ritually abused client, had got his name—from his job. Those children who steadfastly refuse to rape or kill must watch other people do it more violently and are told it is their fault that the victim suffered so much. "Soldier" parts undergo behavioral conditioning to kill or harm without thinking. Military/political and organized crime groups train kids as assassins.

Shaming of victim-perpetrators

After forced perpetration, the perpetrators shame, humiliate, and belittle the children, telling them they are evil. "You are one of us/ Satan's child/evil/a killer/a rapist/an evil witch." "You are a child of the devil and belong only to the coven and the devil." "No one but us will ever want you." "God hates you." "You are going to hell, and your only choice is to be hurt or to hurt others there." "You [especially 'demon' or 'demonized' parts] will harm anyone you get close to; you have special powers that can destroy people's lives." "If you remember any of this, you will remember that you did these evil things." A part is given the job of making the person remember evil acts in which they have been made to participate. In ordinary life, perpetrator group members, especially those in the child's family, attribute anything bad that happens to the child's evil intent.

"Possession"

Are survivors demon-possessed?

Of course not. The abuser groups teach about the guy in the red suit and his minions as if they are literal physical beings. They speak as if demons are bacteria that can be introduced into people's bodies through a mechanical method. That is a childish view, and it is taught to children. "Demons" and "devils" in a survivor are usually small child parts, split off at ages three to five, costumed and taught to make demon sounds by an adult-sized demon impersonator. (Chapter 4 has more details.)

In my opinion, evil is very real, but it does not work in this manner. It requires a free choice to do evil, and a coerced, tortured, terrified child is not making a free choice.

When I first engaged in this work, I tried ordering demon parts to leave the client I was working with. It resulted in those parts hiding and feeling unwanted by me. In another system, the supposedly demonic parts ranged in age up to thirteen and had been given important jobs in the personality system. They were strong cooperators in the healing process. If I had tried to oust them, that client's healing would have stopped.

What about "human spirits"?

Some survivors have parts within them who purport to be the spirits of dead and/or living people. I spent a long time talking with one of my first clients' mother spirit, who talked about her life as if she were actually his mother. Another of my first survivor clients had a part who believed herself to be the survivor's mother; the "mother" part was herself multiple, containing all the actual mother's alter personalities. These "human spirits" are deliberately created introjects—insider parts split off by abusers and usually given the names of those abusers. They often have important responsibilities in the personality system, and oversee other parts, making sure those parts do their jobs. Just as with "demons," if you banish them or lock them away, your survivor client will not be able to fully heal or to undo important programs.

What about ghosts and spirits?

"Ghosts" and other incorporeal entities in a survivor are parts who were led to believe they do not belong to the body (using drugs and stage magic). Sometimes they represent suicide programs (internal homicide)—"Kill this traitor's body." Sometimes they hold knowledge that they supposedly can't disclose because they believe they can't speak. Sometimes they check up on and discipline the system leaders. You won't get to these for a long time; they are hidden. It's important to prove to them that they are in the body. (See Chapter 4.)

Hearing the voice of Jesus or God

Some survivors hear the voice of Jesus or God. It may be simply a playback of a memory involving a person who dressed up as Jesus or God. There will be insiders who have the job of playing this memory back. Or, like a "human spirit," it may be a part who believes that Jesus or God is its name, and it has to say the things the man in the Jesus or God costume used to say. It will give the survivor messages the perpetrator group wants them to hear and obey and believe—false messages. Survivors should not obey instructions from this kind of voice. Instead, they need to talk with it as they would with any other internal voice, recognizing it is a child or teenage part of them. I am not saying that believers cannot communicate with God. I am saying that this is not the way God communicates; it is a deception put into victims by the organized perpetrator groups.

How does evil really work?

Since long before I started to work with survivors of these abuses, I wanted to understand the interface between the psychological, biological, and spiritual in the human mind. This work has, I believe, given me some insights that satisfy my desire to understand.

What are good and evil?

Evil works through temptation and free choice. I believe the nature of good and evil are well summarized in the Golden Rule, which in its simplest form is "Treat others the way you would like them to treat you." The Golden Rule is found in all the major religions. The earliest version is attributed to Confucius: "What you do not want done to yourself, do not do to others." The Buddha is quoted as saying "Since to others, to each one for himself, the self is dear, therefore let him who desires his own advantage not harm another." If we imagine ourselves in the body of the other person, what it would be like to be them, we can see what will help them or harm them. Jesus was quoting Moses (Lev. 19:18) when he told his followers to "Love your neighbor as yourself." Note that he did not say *instead* of yourself. Christians have been mistaken about this for centuries. We now know that self-love is a good thing, and self-esteem helps people have the confidence to help others and make positive contributions to society.

Doing wrong is, simply, violating the Golden Rule. We all do this sometimes, and our conscience tells us that we have done something wrong, to give us the opportunity to put things right. Of course, guilt may also arise when we do something that other people (especially adults, when we are children) have told us is wrong. But this guilt is different from the genuine awareness that we have harmed another. Victims who have been forced to do evil know the difference. Real evildoers choose to violate the Golden Rule repeatedly. The more a person does do this, the less empathy and compassion they have. They have to dissociate their capacity to feel what someone else feels in order to take such actions. Some perpetrators seem to be genuinely evil and perhaps are possessed by evil. But this is a result of the choices they made, not because some adults put demons in them when they were helpless children. Some victims choose to become active perpetrators when given the choice; others choose not to. I believe that most perpetrators in mind-controlling groups were themselves victims who were given choices. Some of them, those who did not become "conscious," chose obedience in order to protect their siblings or children. Others, those who become major perpetrators and group leaders, responded positively to the temptation to have power over others offered them by the perpetrator groups. Conscious perpetrators in these groups (see Chapter 3) are in love with evil. Ritually abused people, when they choose evil, are given the opportunity to do great damage, and pass on their evil to others.

Temptation

Temptation is what we experience when we must make a choice whether or not to heed the Golden Rule. It is repeated yielding to temptation that destroys the soul. This is a primary objective of Satanic and Luciferian groups. They know that all their trappings and tricks mask the real choice about good and evil.

The choices that lead to evil are the same within and outside Satanism. The truly evil takes control of us when we repeatedly yield to what is commonly known as sin—envy, lust for power, control, cruelty, or sexual sadism. Or the simpler lust for material possessions or status at the expense of others. It is an addiction.

Some abusers, not only within organized perpetrator groups but in situations of domestic violence and interpersonal bullying, have had experience of victimization and choose to avoid being victims again by becoming perpetrators, making the other person feel the powerlessness and shame that they do not want to feel again. Harvey Schwartz, in his wonderfully clarifying book *The Alchemy of Wolves and Sheep*, speaks of the motivation of the perpetrator: "The perpetrator evacuates intolerable feelings into the victim's mind and body ... The essence of perpetration is objectification and the systematic undermining of the victim's sense of agency" (2013, p. 109). He quotes Alford in *What Evil Means to Us* (1997, p. 58): "Evil is the attempt to inflict one's doom on others, becoming doom, rather than living subject to it."

Schwartz points out that "The potential for perpetration festers in any environment rife with petty behavior, lies, gossip, objectification or demonization of others, self-absorption, greed, competition, and personal betrayal. ... Not only when under the thumb of child abusing groups, but in churches, universities, places where we all live" (p. 110).

There may or may not be powerful forces of evil that can take over people, pushing or luring them with the temptation to do evil. But if so, they are not the creatures that perpetrator groups purport to insert into helpless children. And they don't just take over a person without the person's consent. Evil is an addiction that gains progressive control over a human mind if the person repeatedly violates the Golden Rule by giving in to the temptation to do harm for personal gain or to avoid personal loss or subjection. We see evil in executives of oil companies who know they are warming the atmosphere and in executives of cigarette and opioid companies who know they are poisoning their customers. We see it in domestic tyrants who apply their power to harm helpless family members and in dictators who destroy the lives of those under their rule. We see it in those victims of organized abuse who choose to join the perpetrators of their own free will. Abuser groups attempt to control their victims to the point that the victims have no choice, no mind of their own. However, some victims, even though their brains split off numerous parts, are successful in resisting such control and refusing, at great personal cost, to become what the perpetrators want.

Guilt, shame, and forgiveness

Moral injury

Moral injury is the damage done to our conscience or moral compass when we perpetrate, witness, or fail to prevent acts that transgress our own moral beliefs, values, or ethical code of conduct. It can lead to serious distress, depression, and suicidality. It is damage done to the soul, the essence of a person. A very young part of one of my clients explained that "It hurts my '*me*.'"

All our clients who are victims of these perpetrator groups have experienced severe moral injury. The perpetrators make sure that their victims believe they (the victims) have deliberately engaged in evil acts, even when they have not done so. Just being present in such a situation can make a person feel utterly contaminated and unworthy. Our clients have been forced to make "lesser of two evils" choices involving harm to others. The horror of coming to know about these choices is extreme. They failed to save others. They may have allowed one victim to be harmed to prevent harm to another they loved more.

Things you can say to a survivor client to counter the abusers' accusation that they are evil:

- Being forced to do something evil feels horrible, but it is the person who forced the victim to do it who is evil, not the victim who was forced. It is no more the fault of the person whose hand held the knife than it is the fault of the knife itself.
- Making a lesser-of-two-evils choice feels horrible, but it is often an act of mercy and kindness, to avoid prolonged suffering for the victim, rather than genuinely evil.
- Most survivors wish they had been the one who died instead of the one who was forced to live and do the abusers' bidding.
- The costumes and fake demons have nothing to do with genuine evil.
- Putting a "demon" in a child doesn't work; it only splits off a new human part who might be taught it is a demon. Perpetrators don't actually have the ability to command demons. Having such a part does not make a child evil.
- The people who direct the international perpetrator networks are not themselves deceived by the trappings. They know these are lies and tricks.

Things you can say to a survivor client about guilt and shame:

- Truly evil people do not feel guilty for what they do. If you feel guilty, it means you still have an inner core of goodness.
- Much of your shame comes from being told it was your fault when some person or creature was harmed.

- If someone bigger and stronger was using your hands to do that harm, it is not your fault.
- If someone else did that harm and told you that your energy was responsible, that is a lie.
- If you were given a forced choice of the lesser of two evils, this does not make you evil.

Things you can say to a survivor client about accountability and remorse:

- It is important not to cut off parts of you who did bad things either because they were forced to or because they didn't understand that those things were bad.
- It is important to forgive parts of you who are truly sorry.
- We all sometimes make the wrong choice and need to be forgiven.
- The mistakes we make do not define who we are.
- Some survivors have parts who have done bad things, such as harmed children, without realizing these things were bad or that the children felt pain. If victim parts of you share how they feel with the parts of you who did those bad things, the parts who did the harm will begin to feel empathy and remorse.

Forgiveness

When a client says to me about a part of them, "Get rid of that part," I reply, "I can't get rid of any part, but I can help them to change." This is the truth. We must never help parts of a person to be in conflict with one another. The parts who appeared loyal to the perpetrators probably saved the person's life and suffered just as greatly as the parts who resisted. Parts need to forgive one another. It also helps some victims to realize that their mother was coerced into abandoning and abusing them in order to save their life, if this is the case. They can soften towards her.

Forgiveness of perpetrators is another matter. Anger and hatred are signs of recovery in survivors, signs that they finally believe they have worth and do not deserve what was done to them. Too many therapists push for premature forgiveness of perpetrators without recognizing the magnitude of the harm that was done. Just because someone is a family member doesn't mean their victim should forgive that person. Only if someone is truly remorseful and genuinely wants to change should the victim forgive that person. Even then, the victim does not have to have that person in their life.

Near-death experiences of victims

A child victim who became my client temporarily died as a result of abuse by her mother. She had a "near-death experience" including a life review in which she learned that the acts of forced evil were not judged as true evil but small acts of petty meanness or unkindness were judged to be evil. Another child victim died while the "Satan's ghost" part was in the front. Unexpectedly, he ("Satan's ghost") found himself being welcomed into a beautiful place, not the hell that he expected. His forced identity didn't matter. He was a hurt child being accepted by the goodness of the afterlife. I have told clients about these experiences of others like them, to reassure them that they are still acceptable. Such near-death experiences are not uncommon among our clients.

Making meaning of the abuse experience

We must face an important fact, which is that God does NOT rescue victims of these abuses or of the Holocaust and other atrocities. Even if we believe in God, we must conclude that God does not micromanage people's lives.

For those of us (and our clients) who want to believe in God, how can we believe that God is all-good, and all-powerful, but these atrocities happen?

I remember reading an essay online arguing that the following three assertions cannot all be true, so when people are struggling to make sense of suffering, they must let go of one of these beliefs: (1) Evil and suffering exist and are real, (2) God is all good, and (3) God is all powerful.

Some people deny the reality of evil and suffering

Some people, even people who courageously bear witness to and work to ease suffering, struggling to make sense of the fact of evil in a world made by a good God, let go of the belief that evil and suffering are real. This is done by asserting that the suffering accomplishes some greater good. You may not realize that you are denying the reality of evil and suffering, but certain statements commonly used show that this is the case.

Here are some statements I have heard made repeatedly.

"Everything happens for a reason"—Whose reason? What reason could be strong enough to justify these events?

"The suffering was necessary to teach a lesson"—This belief makes perpetrators instruments of goodness. It negates the reality and severity of evil.

"Suffering is your karma, payback for a previous life"—To interpret the concept of karma in this way implies that the universe is just and good and that atrocities are necessary and even instruments of healing and purification. It blames the victims.

"What doesn't kill you makes you stronger"—It is true that some people develop extra strength after going through abuse experiences. But it is not the atrocities that made them strong. Those experiences only revealed their inner strength and that of their helpers. Many people are not strengthened but crushed by such experiences and never recover.

No matter what your belief system, I think that using these rationales for suffering diminish the experience of survivors.

Other people choose to deny the existence of a good God

Other people let go of the belief that there is a God who is all good. Here is a quote from Elie Wiesel, Holocaust survivor and prolific writer:

> There is no hope, no comfort, no meaning-making; but there is a survivor's speaking of the evil endured, telling the story, and asserting that there is meaning in telling the story in order to fulfill his promise to bear witness on behalf of those "turned to smoke" so that their story, the horror of their truth, the desecration of their tormenters who not only killed them but also intended to erase their very existence, would not be turned to smoke and lost forever too.

People who take this view speak no platitudes, pretend no happy endings, do no whitewashing of the agony of surviving and the ambivalence of living. They challenge those who stand by and do nothing, and those who hide behind their "neutrality" as "spectators" and "observers." This is a valid choice in dealing with the challenge of making meaning. If a person with this view believes there is an all-powerful God, living can become a protest against Him for His moral corruption. What kind of a God could be responsible for such things? Others may choose atheism, which does not mean negating goodness but choosing to live a good life in the absence of a God who designs everything.

Some people believe that a good God exists but is not all-powerful

A third option, one which is quite valid in the face of evil, is to believe that if there is a God, his power has been limited by the laws of nature that he has created and the necessity of human free will. Good and evil would be meaningless if we were all robots who had no free choice, and if God "stacked the cards" to abrogate the laws of nature whenever things were going to go wrong.

I think that if there is a loving God, that God would suffer with victims rather than side with evil or do nothing. Perhaps God, if He exists, is at every victim's core, giving them moral strength whenever they exercise their free will by choosing not to be like the abusers, whenever they choose kindness and compassion over hatred and power. Just as those who choose evil can become progressively more evil over time, those who choose good, choose to love others and treat others with kindness even at personal expense, can become progressively more good, regardless of their belief systems about the supernatural.

Another well-known Holocaust survivor, Viktor Frankl, founded a school of psychotherapy that describes a search for life's meaning as the central human motivational force. Every human being, including those who go through these horrendous abuses, searches for the meaning of their life. We therapists, just like our clients, engage in this search, and both we and our clients must face the dilemma imposed by the presence and power of evil. Whether you are an atheist or a believer in a good God, you are engaged in the struggle between good and evil. It is important that we therapists not impose our own chosen beliefs on our clients, who have had their minds and their entire lives controlled by others. They deserve to find their own meaning, just as we do.

CHAPTER 10

Healing for our clients and ourselves

Effects of the abuse on survivors

Deprivation of normal experiences

Our survivor clients, for the most part, never had parents who didn't abuse them, parents with whom they could form bonds of trust. Family meant abuse and neglect and torture. They never had emotional security. They never had physical safety and a chance for healthy development with adequate food and drink and sleep. Their basic needs were not met. They had no chance for healthy brain development. Instead, their brain circuitry was systematically split to produce programmed robotic parts. They never had normal childish enjoyment and play. They were never permitted to have true friends, except, in many cases, only one, who was then killed. They never had a chance to relax rather than be in constant overdrive. They didn't have an education that developed their true abilities and interests. They were never given the opportunity to know and meet their own needs and develop purpose. They were denied independent thought. They never had a chance for the healthy development of sexuality in loving relationships. Yet so many of the courageous survivors that we have come to know are determined to persist in the healing process, to refuse to become like their abusers, to become themselves. We cannot help but wonder what we would have done in the same situation.

Survivors have experienced many losses. For many, their only childhood friend was killed. Their childhood pets were killed. Those whose families were abusers have had to suffer the permanent loss of family in order to heal. Most feel isolated from people around them, who don't and usually can't understand what their lives have been like, so even if they have achieved freedom they feel alone. Many have spent years with therapists who don't understand their condition or their history or how to help them heal. Older survivors no longer have the chance to live a fulfilling life (although some have made tremendous achievements later in life).

Physical effects of the abuse

The Adverse Childhood Experiences (ACE) study showed that most severe and chronic illnesses are more common based on how many kinds of adverse childhood experiences the victim suffered. Survivors of ritual abuse and mind control have every kind of adverse experience, multiple times over. The abuse has also had direct physical effects. Most victims have chronic inflammation and pain, with injuries to the neck, spine, joints, vagina/urethra, anus/rectum, and abdomen/large intestine. Chronic severe headaches are common, as are sleep difficulties and consequent chronic exhaustion. Many victims have had repeated concussions, which can affect the functioning of the brain. Although some physical symptoms are body memories that can be relieved with memory work, others are injuries that cannot be rectified. This is very hard for survivors to live with.

Healing tasks

I have focused so far on survivors' undoing the deliberate programming in order to regain control of their own lives. The goal of this is becoming one person, a single self, or a cooperative system of selves with internal conflict significantly reduced and no internal punishment. But there are other important tasks for full healing: recovering and expressing emotions, grieving for losses and deprivations, developing friendships, overcoming shame, and developing self-esteem.

Emotional healing

Our many emotions are normal, healthy responses to what is happening to us. Emotions exist to tell us about our needs, so that we can take action to get those needs met. Just as hunger tells us we need food, and physical pain tells us we need to pay attention to a medical problem, loneliness tells us we need interpersonal connection, and anger tells us we need to work hard to overcome an obstacle or stop an injustice.

For victims of mind control, emotions were either prohibited and locked away in emotion-holding infant parts or deliberately put into specific parts for the abusers' use (for example, anger for perpetration and despair for suicidality). "Booby traps" installed by abusers involve despair, feeling unloved, with the emotions of parts who are made to believe that they live in cages or in hell or in the garbage pit. Such insiders may see the whole world as like their abuse scenarios. They need to be rescued by other insiders. Even though working through the training memories helps connect emotions from the past to the events they belong with, there are usually still leftover emotions that need to be expressed and released. Anger needs healthy expression through such means as making a noise, singing and shouting, writing poetry, memoirs, and books to tell what happens and to help others, as well as putting experiences and feelings into art. Sadness needs to be cried out with someone who cares, overcoming the terrifying "don't cry" training. We therapists can facilitate this process.

Grieving

As awareness of what has happened grows, survivors must grieve, one loss at a time: the loss of illusions about their life, as well as all the other losses and deprivations they have endured. How can we assist them in this process?

Your client needs a compassionate witness who doesn't underreact or overreact. Don't dismiss or minimize the depth of your client's horrendous experiences and losses. Don't point out all the good things when they are talking about the bad things. Don't give answers. Just "sit with a shattered soul." Your client must grieve about what happened to them, and you must grieve about what happened to them and the reality that such things happen to many innocent children. However, it is important not to catch your client's depression and despair and hypervigilance. Allow the client's feelings to come into you but recognize they are not your own. "Lean in but don't fall in." Seek knowledgeable supervision and peer support.

Survivor Wendy Hoffman in 2022 wrote for her presentation on self-esteem for Survivorship and SmartNews (see their websites):

> Grief has always been meant to be shared. Religions of all sorts have arranged for people to sit together and share loss. In these mind control cults, however, grief and the parts that hold it are isolated, without comfort, or communion, or anything that will replace the loss.

We can listen. We can acknowledge that even though we can't understand the enormity of what has happened to them, they can be our teachers, and we can be with them as they recover.

One sad thing about being a therapist is that we cannot be there forever in our clients' lives. We cannot meet their every need, even though we may long to do so. Most survivors have no true friends, as those have not been allowed or are dead. Survivors need to develop friendships with good people who care about them. Sadly, most ordinary people cannot tolerate hearing and knowing about the abuses our clients have endured. But some can. One true friend can make an enormous difference. Some survivors may actually find a safe, loving, and supportive spouse. So, we must encourage our clients to reach out and find friends who are not plants or handlers.

Helping survivors develop self-esteem

Many if not most of us grow up with parents who set conditions of worth on us. We are acceptable to them only if we measure up to certain standards, such as being perfect, being the best, or being "good" and obedient. We internalize those conditions of worth, and therefore develop vulnerable self-esteem. Low and fluctuating self-esteem is characteristic of many people, not just those who were severely abused as children. Depending on our conditions of worth, our self-esteem can go up and down. If we succeed or are praised, we may have inflated self-esteem (conceit), but then when we fail or are criticized, we lose self-esteem and feel humiliated. When we accept ourselves as we are (with idiosyncrasies and weaknesses and mistakes and failures) because we are learning, growing human beings, we can laugh at ourselves, and we can forget ourselves and concentrate on the other people we are with and what they need. However, if our self-esteem is based on conditional love for ourselves, we are unable to do this. True self-esteem means simply esteeming the self as it is.

This is in itself a sufficient challenge for most of us, but mind control survivors were not permitted any mistakes as children. Falling short of perfection led to severe punishment. A survivor therapist wrote: "I get a lot of second-guessing happening in me after I say or do anything where Inside picks it all to pieces and speculates if I was too vivacious, quiet, odd, intense, boring, interesting, showed other people up, etc. Can't win." Many people who have not been abused but have lived with conditional parental love go through this, but it is especially strong if someone has been exposed to mind control. Perpetrators believe that reducing their victims' self-esteem is a necessary condition of mind control. So, an important part of healing for our clients is learning to accept their weaknesses and mistakes, and even laughing about them. We can set an example of this.

Wendy Hoffman wrote to survivors:

> Programmers—all mind-controlled people have programmers —make you think that you deserve nothing in life and are just a marionette on a tight string and a means for your controllers to get what they want … Programmers take an event that you innocently participated in, change the facts so that you think you did something bad and feel guilty. They show you fabricated pictures to "prove" your guilt. They want you to go through life thinking you are a bad person.

It is not our fault that we were born into generational cults. It is not our fault that we had parents who were prisoners themselves and could not or were not willing to help their children. It is not our fault that mind control has reached new heights and is hard to decipher, hard but not impossible. All that is reason to respect yourself, value yourself, cherish yourself and fight. Fight for the right to be who you are. Not someone else's creation of you but who you really are on your own. There are pleasures in life, the pleasure of sleep, satisfying hunger, walking in the sun, shade, clean air. And the greatest pleasure, discovering who you are.

I can't stress enough how we were not treated as people, how our bodies were considered objects to abuse, to use for perpetrators' selfish desires. A part of you may think they were right, justified. That misinformed part may be buried deep inside but may be there feeding your thoughts and beliefs. They were not right. They are wrong. You are human and alive. Your body is part of you. It deserves respect, it is worthwhile, precious. It has integrity.

After much healing, she wrote:

The new me looks back and feels love and tenderness for these old parts who no longer have to exist and perform. The strings of these marionettes are clipped, the chains of the slaves broken. They are free now. They reach out their arms to the new emerging self, the new emerging self reaches out their arms to them. They love one another. The essential is to love yourself, to comfort yourself, to be true to yourself. For many of us who have to leave our families behind, the self is the new family. Be kind, accepting, stick by yourself. It is what you have now.

As therapists, we can help by encouraging survivor clients to think for themselves, to refuse the internal messages of blame and shame, to forgive themselves for things they were made to do, and for being imperfect human beings. We can encourage them to love and accept the person they are rather than trying to live up to anyone else's standards.

Some steps in learning to accept yourself are identifying and letting go of your conditions of worth, choosing to be your true self rather than what other people want, taking charge of your own life, allowing yourself mistakes and failures, and allowing yourself to receive from others what they have to give. It is particularly hard for survivors of mind-controlling abuses to receive help from others (including therapists) after lives in which every supposed helper turned out to be an abuser. Survivors can start with small things, allowing a neighbor to help clear the driveway or bring food when they are sick.

Integration? Fusion?

The healing process may take years, not necessarily all in therapy. Integration is a gradual process, usually involving small groups of parts joining together when they process the memories that split them apart in the first place. I do not believe in planned or forced fusion of parts. Forced fusions will traumatize front parts with unresolved memories and will come apart.

Abusers have told child parts that integration means their death, so they may be terrified of this natural process in which no part dies, it just becomes part of a larger whole. It helps to have integrated parts let unintegrated parts know what it is like for them to be an amalgamation of two or more parts or sections. Joining of parts happens naturally when memories they share are resolved. When parts are ready to integrate, nothing can stop them.

It's possible for all parts within a particular subsystem to fully integrate while another subsystem remains untouched. Ongoing harassment targets the untouched subsystem. Therapy can last for many years, and the healing process is lifelong, and continues after therapy is finished. I think that all of us who are growing human beings are undergoing an integration process, learning to accept and bring together all aspects of ourselves.

Intimidation of therapists

Some perpetrator groups engage in attempts to intimidate therapists. My first recognition of intimidation came when a police detective came uninvited to my office to tell me that when people had reported ritualistic things to the police, "We have methods to make them admit they made it all up." When I later met with police officers from all the local police forces, trying to get police involved regarding serious crimes reported by my clients, I was offered that same detective, and I refused to work with him.

There was a discussion of this issue in the Organized and Extreme Abuse discussion group of the ISST-D. A therapist reported that a drone flew over her back yard, and that her ritually abused client had told her that the abuser group often flew drones over her home. She asked whether she should be worried. Amy Connor responded:

> In my years of working with this population intimidation has come in many forms, from survivors telling me that insect nan- otechnology is in my home, to the "white van" intimidation, to weaponry in the session room, to finally the disclosure of what orders and threats had been given, to a military chopper flying through my yard so low the ground trembled. These are just a few.

Susan Pease Banitt wrote:

> BIG DUH: going up against organized crime and government projects means pushback—especially when we are successful … They know who you are. They know who everybody is doing this work. The good news is you're not paranoid. The bad news is you're not paranoid! … They can only tip their hand so far with- out us networking with each other or becoming too "real" in the eyes of the public. Take reasonable precautions. Get the highest levels of insurance and licensure defense.

She also wrote:

> It makes sense they are using drones now—cheaper and less obtrusive than the old school helicopter/light plane surveillance that older patients of mine reported. That being said, I'd go out and give that drone the finger—consider that a clinical bound- ary setting intervention.

Another discussion member wrote:

> If it were me, I think I might make a report to law enforcement, with a photo of the drone if I could catch one, and state that I believe it was sent by people who are endangering one of my clients, but that I cannot disclose the identity of the client or the perpetrators I suspect for client confidentiality and client safety reasons, but that if any harm were to come to me, that information will be held by my legal representative and turned over to the police at such time. The fact that I made such a report might find its way back to the perpetrators and make them think twice about continuing to harass me.

There was also discussion of technology for spying on therapy. Bas Kremer wrote:

> There are of course specialized apps to monitor or eavesdrop on someone via his or her smartphone. Even in a standard app like WhatsApp it is easy to turn on your location and make it specifically visible where you are. These types of apps will no doubt be used, including by network loyal parts inside our clients. It is also always a good idea to ask your client in case of ongoing abuse or doubt about it, to physically switch off your smartphone completely [in the therapy session].

Some of the groups also engage in attempted psychic attacks on therapists. Whether or not we believe it is real, we should be aware that these groups do use their psychic adepts to attack us, our mental health, and our physical health. I found many strange coincidences happening whenever I was about to do a presentation about these abuses, from lost luggage to a new dogsitter stealing my dog. If you believe psychic attacks can harm you, you may want to find a way to put up a boundary. I like to imagine a mirror surrounding me, facing outwards, so anything psychic sent at me gets bounced back to the sender. (Of course, I don't know whether it works.)

I have sometimes noticed intimidation attempts by perpetrator groups coming to me via clients, and I engaged for years in a kind of war with the local Serpents cult. I have no doubt they were trying to assess me and what I might react to. There was the message "We know where you live," conveyed by a client showing up on my birthday on my lawn with a dozen pink flamingos, a big sign giving my name and age, a big smile, and a camera to take a picture of us together with all this paraphernalia. There was the message "We are going to kill you in a very unpleasant manner," coming through that client's recounting the threat to me in gory detail as it had been told to her. That client was not herself trying to intimidate me on behalf of the cult, but parts of her were relaying the messages the cult had given her for me. I needed to stay strong and caring with her, and not back off the work with her and other clients.

Amy Connor wrote to our discussion group:

> It is important they feel my solidity, security, and steady nature so that the whole system can assess what space I am capable of holding with them. If I recognize intimidation tactics, I refuse to be intimidated. This takes a progressive calm sense of introspection, reasoning, planning, and acting (because what safety steps are possible need to be considered) ... I will always be checking in with myself internally about my own state of regulation because the world we live in is the world we live in and we are important too.

Do they kill therapists? I know of two possible such murders, both back in the early years of my work with this population, one an apparent suicide, another a boat capsizing. I did have my car's brake cable snap twice within a year. (My car was not an automatic, so I managed to brake by using the clutch.) In those years (the early 1990s), they did sometimes poison therapists with pesticide, not to kill them but to intimidate them. I experienced this once at a conference. I think the groups are much more cautious now. We must assess the degree of risk we are willing to tolerate and take precautions.

Therapists' vicarious traumatization

I wish I lived in the world I lived in when I was a child, where children played on the street and (as far as I knew) neighbors looked after them safely. I wish I lived in the world I (thought I) lived in as a young adult, where God looked after those who tried to live good lives and had faith, and we could trust Him not to send us more than we could bear. Climate change and the pandemic and the Ukraine and Israel-Hamas wars have made previously secure people afraid.

But long before the recent world events that have cracked open humanity's denial, I had begun to know through my work the evil that some human beings engage in, which has festered underneath the surface and is now leading to disastrous events. Through this work I learned that what society knows as abuse is just the top layer of what goes on. I learned that there is really a conspiracy, more than one, but not the ones the conspiracy theorists publicize. I learned that people do the most horrible things within families, and especially to infants and little children, at the most important stage of life. I learned that the extent of human capacity for evil is profound, and that this holocaust continues, focusing on children. I learned that leaders of society are a crucial part of abuser groups. I learned that to produce programmed spies and assassins, law enforcement and countries' militaries engage in hidden torture, even of children. What I learned made me profoundly sad. And angry enough to pursue helping survivors and supporting those who have the courage to treat them.

On the Organized and Extreme Abuse discussion group of the ISST-D, Lysa Toye wrote:

> It makes sense that we are marked by the work. The deeper I go into learning about extreme abuse, the more important it becomes for me to actively practice joy and space in my body and the somatic knowing of love and connection and ease, just so I can hold my growing knowing that the world is full of unspeakable harms, and that sexual harms are so commonplace that they feel like the fabric of society and our intergenerational shaping, the same as misogyny and racism and colonialism and war and all the forms of dominance and subjugation—and— that there is love and goodness and possibility for repair.

Many therapists are overwhelmed. When I required my supervised associates to read Wendy Hoffman's first memoir, *The Enslaved Queen*, one man said he had never heard of such profound evil. All of them had difficulty reading it. We are overwhelmed by the darkness and the horror of what has happened to our clients. Many therapists refuse to do this work, passing such clients on to those few who stay in the field, making the excuse of ignorance. Yet survivors need us very badly. There are very few therapists who specialize in this clientele, and some of these are plants, taught by the perpetrator groups to close down their clients' memories and prevent their healing. If a reader of this book is a plant therapist, I encourage you to learn from the book, work privately on your own healing, and try to find ways to help your clients while appearing to be doing the job you were planted to do. You too are a victim.

We experience vicarious traumatization from empathizing with persons who from birth onward have suffered in "the hidden Holocaust" (a term suggested by a survivor), and from seeing them abreact the abuse in front of our eyes. We must live with the awareness that persons we have come to care about are being tortured on an ongoing basis and may be harassed for years and years. We know that many such clients, especially older ones, may not be able to achieve a high quality of life even after therapy, and some may not even want to try. We may be overwhelmed by the necessarily long duration of the work (even though it also allows a deep meaningful relationship), the complexity of the work (which challenges our brains), and the lack of sufficient clear guidelines on how to proceed (which also provides room for creativity).

Vicarious traumatization is not the same as burnout. Burnout comes from working too hard without a break. Vicarious traumatization is the effect of really listening to and hearing horrendous stories. It is common in first responders, military personnel who have been in combat, medical personnel in the pandemic, and medical personnel in wars and natural disasters. While we were not physically present when the children who became our clients were tortured, we are resonating with those children when they reenter those memories.

Symptoms of vicariously traumatized therapists

- Lingering feelings of anger, rage, and sadness about our clients' victimization
- Overinvolvement emotionally with victimized clients

- Difficulty in maintaining professional boundaries, overextending ourselves
- Bystander guilt, shame, and self-doubt
- Preoccupation with thoughts about the survivor client outside the work situation
- Horror and rescue fantasies
- Loss of hope, pessimism, cynicism
- Distancing, numbing, detachment, not listening, feeling emotionally numb
- Feeling vulnerable or worrying excessively about dangers and our loved ones' safety
- Irritability, aggressive or explosive outbursts
- Decreased participation in activities we used to enjoy.

We need to monitor ourselves for such symptoms. We do need to feel with our clients, but not let those feelings take over our lives. We must hold on to ourselves and our perspective. It's good to show we feel compassion and sadness (when these are genuine), to let the client see that we care but are not overwhelmed. It's like a parent with an upset child. Don't let their feelings overwhelm you; remain calm and confident but mirror their feelings within your heart or soul.

Strategies to reduce risk to your own mental health

Most information I give here comes from various websites on vicarious traumatization, as well as from online discussions in which I have participated.

Begin with awareness of what is going on with you. Increase your self-observation. Be realistic about what you can accomplish, and help your clients find their own tools for self-care; don't take it all on yourself.

Then there's balance: Balance your caseload with non-victim clients. Take regular breaks and time off. Keep strong boundaries about private time, and limit other trauma exposures, including those online or on television.

Maintain positive experiences, so you won't be overwhelmed by the negative experiences your clients bring to you. Engage in relaxing and self-nurturing activities to look after your physical and mental well-being. Spend time in nature, smell the flowers. Soothe your body through baths, massage, and enjoyable food. Read enjoyable books, watch enjoyable television shows, listen to podcasts. Exercise every day in a way that you enjoy.

Finally, we all need connection. Seek support from colleagues and debrief with peers. As many of your local peers won't understand what you are dealing with, seek out online discussion groups with other therapists treating survivors, which can help you feel understood and supported, as long as confidentiality is maintained. Engage in personal therapy and/or supervision if you need more support, with a therapist who understands what you are dealing with. Spend time with friends outside of work. Spend time petting your pets (as well as playing with them and exercising with them, if they're animals that need exercise). Keep your family relationships healthy by putting aside enough time for your partner and/or children.

Posttraumatic growth: areas of growth

We therapists must recognize that the work traumatizes us, and then look at how we come out of it. The trauma literature talks about post-traumatic growth in various areas: appreciation of life and what we have, deepened relationships with our clients and like-minded peers, new possibilities in life as we move into an area of work that challenges us and forces us to develop strength and creativity, and spiritual change as we have a more realistic approach to life and faith, based on reality, not on wishful thinking or lies we've been told.

How this work is fulfilling

This work has satisfied my need to do *real* psychology and understand how the human brain/mind/psyche/spirit works. It has answered some of my basic questions about the universe. It has allowed and required me to "wing it," be creative, and develop new methods of helping the most grievously wounded. It has been an excellent way to use the gifts I have been given. It has allowed me to contribute to making the world a better place. It has allowed me to form deep connections with some incredible, resilient, and good people, my clients.

For all of us, the knowledge that we have helped someone, that we have done something good, that we have the capacity to help and even to save lives, that our creativity has worked to help someone, is very satisfying. I hope this will be the experience of every therapist who reads this book. And that some of you, and some of your clients (and survivors who also read this book), will contribute to knowledge and expertise in this field.

References

Alford, C. F. (1997). *What Evil Means to Us*. Ithaca, NY: Cornell University Press.

Callow, J. (2012). Building inner community: Living happily without integration. In: A. Miller, *Healing the Unimaginable: Treating Ritual Abuse and Mind Control* (pp. 272–275). London: Karnac.

Callow, J. (2014). How I created my inner community: Living happily without integration. In: A. Miller, *Becoming Yourself: Overcoming Mind Control and Ritual Abuse* (pp. 151–154). London: Karnac.

Centers for Disease Control and Prevention. The CDC-Kaiser Permanente adverse childhood experiences (ACE) study. https://cdc.gov/violence-prevention/aces/about.html (last accessed January 25, 2024).

Extreme Abuse Survey. http://eassurvey.wordpress.com/extreme-abuse-survey-final-results/ (last accessed January 25, 2024).

Farber, S. K. (2018). The relationship of mental telepathy to trauma and dissociation. *Frontiers in the Psychotherapy of Trauma and Dissociation, 1*(2): 267–289.

Fotheringham, T. (2012). Mind control as I experienced it. In: A. Miller, *Healing the Unimaginable: Treating Ritual Abuse and Mind Control* (pp. 74–85). London: Karnac.

Green, A. (2014). Downfall. In: A. Miller, *Becoming Yourself: Overcoming Mind Control and Ritual Abuse* (pp. 298–302). London: Karnac.

Health Resources and Services Administration. National Child Traumatic Stress Network. https://hrsa.gov/behavioral-health/national-child-traumatic-stress-network-nctsn (last accessed January 20, 2024).

Hoffman, W. (2014). *The Enslaved Queen: A Memoir about Electricity and Mind Control*. London: Karnac.

Hoffman, W. (2022). *After Amnesia and During*. Survivorship and SmartNews websites.

Hoffman, W., & Miller, A. (2018). *From the Trenches: A Victim and Therapist Talk about Mind Control and Ritual Abuse*. London: Karnac.

International Society for the Study of Trauma and Dissociation. Treatment Guidelines, Organized and Extreme Abuse special interest group. www.isst-d.org/ (last accessed January 25, 2024).

Katz, S. (2012). A reversed Kabbalah trainer speaks. In: A. Miller, *Healing the Unimaginable: Treating Ritual Abuse and Mind Control* (Chapter 7). London: Karnac.

Miller, A. (2012a). *Healing the Unimaginable: Treating Ritual Abuse and Mind Control*. London: Karnac.

Miller, A. (2012b). Dialogue with the higher-ups. In: R. Vogt (Ed.), *Perpetrator Introjects: Psychotherapeutic Diagnostics and Treatment Models* (pp. 111–132). Kroning, Germany: Asanger.

Miller, A. (2014). *Becoming Yourself: Overcoming Mind Control and Ritual Abuse*. London: Karnac.

Miller, A. (2019). Commentary: Therapeutic neutrality, ritual abuse, and maladaptive daydreaming. *Frontiers in the Psychotherapy of Trauma & Dissociation*, 3(1): 4–11. DOI: 10.46716/ftpd.2019.0018.

Sachs, A. (2012). Boundary modifications in the treatment of people with dissociative disorders: A pilot study. *Journal of Trauma and Dissociation*, 14(2): 159–169.

Schwartz, H. L. (2013). *The Alchemy of Wolves and Sheep: A Relational Approach to Internalized Perpetration in Complex Trauma Survivors*. New York: Routledge.

Sharman, M. (2014). My sexual healing process. In: A. Miller, *Becoming Yourself: Overcoming Mind Control and Ritual Abuse* (pp. 265–271). London: Karnac.

Van der Hart, O., & Nijenhuis, E. (1999). Bearing witness to uncorroborated trauma: The clinician's development of reflective belief. *Professional Psychology: Research and Practice*, 30(1): 37–44.

Index